AIDS: THE HIDDEN AGENDA IN CHILD SEXUAL ABUSE

AIDS: The Hidden Agenda in Child Sexual Abuse

**Chris Bennetts, Mae Brown,
Jane Sloan**

LONGMAN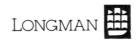

AIDS: THE HIDDEN AGENDA IN CHILD SEXUAL ABUSE

Published by Longman Group UK Ltd, Westgate House, The High,
Harlow, Essex CM20 1YR, UK.
Telephone: (0279) 442601
Fax: (0279) 444501
Telex: 81491 Padlog

First published 1992

**A catalogue record for this book is available from the British
Library**

ISBN 0-582-09825-4

Printed and bound in Great Britain by
Biddles Ltd, Guildford and King's Lynn

Contents

Acknowledgements

The authors would like to acknowledge and thank the following people for their help in the preparation of this book:

Amanda Godfrey and Wendy Wilson for their patience and precision in typing this manuscript; friends and colleagues for their understanding and forbearance while we were struggling with this task.

Chris would particularly like to thank Dr David Miles for his constructive support; Simmy Viinikka and Moira Wilson for their helpful comments on chapter 12, Section 3; and Clive for the countless cups of coffee.

Foreword

The experience of child sexual abuse brings pain and grief to many children every year. More widely it affects families and friends, social groups and neighbourhoods. Professionals working with HIV infection can testify to the similar levels of distress and grief which are aroused where a life-threatening illness is either feared or diagnosed. Both experiences bring with them the possibility of stigma and isolation. Where a child has suffered both abuse and the possibility of infection, a situation arises where the level of feeling and the complexity of the issues make it a formidable challenge to all involved.

In the face of these difficulties, an increasing number of professionals will have to work to find ways of helping children and their families where HIV infection following abuse is either a possibility or a reality. Working across professional boundaries, the authors of this book offer examples of how it is possible to provide a comprehensive and sensitive professional response.

The authors have drawn upon their own practical and direct experience of the issues and set this experience in the context of current knowledge of the field. At the same time they have, very importantly, ensured that the child and his or her understanding of events are a central focus.

This is a difficult and challenging area of work. Not only does the direct work with children call for particular strengths and skills, but the required partnership between different professional groups may demand both initiative and persistence.

Training and preparation of staff is a vital prerequisite if children and their families are to be properly served by the professional community. At the Child Abuse Training Unit, we know that professionals in different disciplines and throughout the UK are currently struggling with these issues. We warmly welcome this book and recommend it to managers, trainers and practitioners.

Helen Armstrong
Child Abuse Training Unit
National Children's Bureau

Introduction

At a recent seminar funded by the Department of Health to allow representatives from the agencies primarily concerned with child protection to look at their area response to multiple abuse situations, the group facilitator raised the issue of HIV/AIDS counselling for the victims.

A social worker present indicated that, in a situation where there were no agreed procedures for dealing with multiple abuse situations, HIV/AIDS counselling was somewhat low on the list of priorities.

A doctor responsible for medically assessing the children who were the victims in a multiple abuse situation, commented that almost the first question asked by the child and the child's parents was about the risk of AIDS.

The answers probably illustrate the gap which exists presently between social workers and health service personnel in considering the implications of AIDS when examining a response to the sexual abuse of children, whether by a single perpetrator or in a multiple abuse situation.

Perhaps an alternative title for this book should be 'Fools Rush In'! The subject of child sexual abuse arouses strong emotions including intense denial. To add to this emotive subject the possibility that professionals may also have to consider HIV infection becomes distinctly taboo. It is bad enough to consider the sexual humiliation and degradation to which children are subjected. To then realise that the activity could be life threatening becomes almost beyond thought.

However, all professionals need to be aware of the psychological, physical and lego-ethical minefield which lies ahead. Not only must professionals dealing with child sexual abuse be aware of the possibility of HIV infection, but HIV counsellors need to understand the impact of child sexual abuse. Fear of AIDS may be the trigger which enables a child to speak of abuse. There will be occasions when an AIDs educator in a school will be the first person to whom a child talks about sexual activity which is abusive. Both sides need to understand the roles and functions of the other and the limitations to those roles. Equally, both sides will need to adapt their work to fit the developmental and emotional status of the individual child. It is with this in mind that this book was planned.

It is an attempt to bring together the knowledge of a social worker, an educationalist and a health worker to outline a response in this situation. As far as it is possible to ascertain, this has not been done before. There are countless books on child development, as well as innumerable tomes on child sexual abuse, together with a growing number of books on HIV/AIDS. There does not appear to be a single book making the connection between all three subjects. A specialist in any of these three subjects would look elsewhere for detailed information on their specialist subject. Basic information is provided to enable professionals to gain sufficient information to respond in a child-centred way in any of the three areas.

Section 1 is an explanation of child development at a level to help not only social workers but also HIV/AIDS counsellors and other health personnel, to respond appropriately to children who have been sexually abused and may also, in the process, have contracted a life threatening illness. It brings these issues together in describing the particular problems encountered by children abused as part of a sex ring.

The second section of the book aims to give those unfamiliar with the response to sexual abuse recommended by the Department of Health — and the problems to that response — a basic understanding of the theory and practice. It also deals with the legislative framework for protecting children.

The third and final section looks at the practicalities of counselling abused children who may have been infected by HIV. It outlines not only the current terminology and state of knowledge of the disease but also the medical and legal issues which must be considered in any counselling situation.

Except when giving specific examples, a conscious effort has been made throughout the book to use non-gender specific language when discussing either abusers or victims.

Statistically, the overwhelming proportion of known abusers are male, and females outnumber males as known victims. On the other hand, many males are victims, and females can also abuse. By adopting the more common terminology which refers to abusers as 'he' and victims as 'she', these sex-role stereotypes are further reinforced, making it the more difficult to keep an open mind when faced with an allegation of sexual abuse.

The authors, although having many years experience of working with both children and adults who have been abused, do not claim a research orientation for this book. It is based on practical experience and the learning acquired, sometimes painfully, through trial and error. It is in acute awareness of those errors that we would like to dedicate this book to all victims of sexual abuse in the hope that in some way it may help make survival less painful for at least a few.

Contributors

Chris Bennetts, MITD is a Senior Health Promotions Officer for AIDS education (Adults). She is presently studying for an MEd in Training and Development at Sheffield University and has also been a Senior Health Promotion Officer in AIDS Education (Young People).

Mae H. Brown, MA, MEd, AFBPsS, CPsychol is a Senior Educational Psychologist working with a local Education Authority with special responsibility for liaison with Social Services. She specialises in assessment and treatment of sexually abused and traumatised children. Previous posts include teacher Senior Education Psychology in Scotland and Tutor to the Dip Ed course at Glasgow University.

Jane C. Sloan, BsocSc, DipPSW, PQSW is a Social Work Consultant (Child Protection) for Cornwall County Council. She has previously worked as a medical social worker for the NSPCC, a teacher/social worker and teacher.

Section 1 DEVELOPMENTAL ISSUES

Introduction

The first three chapters of this section follow a similar format and consider the developmental aspects of children from the preschool years to adolescence with particular reference to children who have been sexually abused. The features of a child's development which are important for social workers and AIDS counsellors to take into consideration are highlighted. It was not the intention to cover all areas of the development of children, but for those who wish to investigate the topic in greater depth, appropriate books are listed in the resources section at the end. Although these chapters indicate what is to be expected in the various age groups, it is important to remember that all children do not progress at the same rate and there is a wide variation in children's skills at any specific age. Those children with special needs develop at a slower rate in some areas and may never attain age appropriate levels. For ease of reference, the chapters have been divided into age groups but many developmental processes are continuous in nature and this should be borne in mind.

Chapter 4 looks at the phenomenon of sex rings and the effects these rings have on victims and their families. When children are subjected to this type of sexual abuse involving offenders who frequently have long histories of sexual assault, they are clearly at increased risk of HIV infection. There is an even greater risk for victims if these acts are committed by paedophiles who have reoffended after a period of imprisonment.

1 Preschool children

Introduction

The preschool years are an exciting stage of development as young children are learning new skills, acquiring language and finding out about themselves and the world they inhabit. However, unless we understand the limitations of this developmental stage and have some knowledge of how a child thinks and understands the world, we may be in danger of making false assumptions and misinterpreting what the child is trying to communicate. In one sense young children are straightforward in their responses but in another they are very different creatures from the adult or the older child. We must, therefore, take into account the developmental perspective if we wish to communicate successfully with young children.

Young children as thinkers

It is very tempting for adults to assume that young children have the same thought processes as ourselves, albeit less sophisticated. However, nothing could be further from the truth. Trying to understand how children think has fascinated psychologists for many years. Piaget, a famous Swiss psychologist, was the first to study the patterns of development which are common to all children and he named the period from two to six years the 'preoperational stage of cognitive development'. In this stage, children are able to use symbols such as language in their thinking, but they have not yet acquired the ability to think in a logical manner.

Children of varying ages were watching an adult placing a number of different coloured counters in a bag, then pulling out one counter at a time. Before every draw, the adult asked the children to predict what colour would be drawn. 'Blue' said a ten year old, 'blue hasn't come up for a while.' 'Red' said one four year old confidently, and when asked why 'cos I like red'.

This example illustrates clearly the differences in the thinking processes of the 10 year old and the four year old. The preschool child is thinking from his own point of view and is not using what adults would call logic. It is most important for the adult to understand that young children think that the world revolves around them and they assume that others see the world from their point of view. Piaget (1954) named this quality of the young child's thinking *'Egocentrism'.* The preschool child has great difficulty in understanding the other person's perspective even if that other person is another child.

> Mary had been looking forward to starting school for a long time and was highly delighted when the great day arrived. At the school gate, Mary's mother met a friend whose little girl was also starting school and Mary was instructed to take Jean's hand and look after her. At lunchtime Mary came home and her mother asked if she had enjoyed school. She was surprised when Mary complained about having to look after Jean who had cried all morning. 'Why is she crying?' demanded Mary, and when her mother tried to explain that Jean was probably upset because she missed her mother, Mary was astonished. She was quite convinced that because she was excited at the idea of starting school, Jean would be also. It was beyond Mary's ability to understand that someone else might view the experience in a different manner.

Young children's thinking is based on their own views and feelings and it does not relate to those of other people. When Peter closes his eyes in a game of hide and seek, he assumes that because he cannot see you, you cannot see him. As children of this age are unaware of what effect their actions will have on others, they do not concern themselves with what others think. Saying what they think out loud in a spontaneous manner can often cause great embarrassment to adults. Although egocentric thought is typical of the young child, we must remember that as adults, we never completely lose the ability to think from our own point of view. As King and Yuille (1987) state, 'the real danger of egocentrism may be the egocentricity of the adult who is unable to appreciate fully the child's perspective in an interview'.

Young children have very limited experience and understanding of the world and if they are being sexually abused they accept this as 'how things are', especially if other needs are being met, i.e. for affection and attention. When you are a child your expectation depends on what you have experienced. How is the young child to know that the game daddy plays with her is not played by all daddies? Guilt is not an issue for the preschool child although they may complain if an activity hurts. This is understandably the age when most disclosures of abuse are accidental as children are not aware of the significance of what they are saying. The abuse may become so much a part of their world that they see no need to tell another adult unless they are frightened or hurt by the experience, and the only way we may be able to detect what is happening is through the child's behaviour and play. It is essential that the adult who is interviewing young children or interpreting their verbal accounts of sexual abuse, attempts to see the situation from the child's perspective, as what is significant detail for the child may not be significant for the adult.

As young children see themselves at the centre of the world, it is all too easy for them to misinterpret what they see. They believe that objects have the same feelings and wishes they have, a characteristic Piaget (1929) labelled 'Animism'. Small children will often refer to an inanimate object such as a chair as 'naughty' because they bumped into it. This confusion of real and unreal is reinforced by children's literature where toys and animals are portrayed as being able to speak and having feelings and wishes with which children can identify. Moreover, we systematically teach our children about Santa Claus, the Tooth Fairy and Easter Bunny as part of our culture, and they are portrayed on television alongside real events: 'Children are prone to live in a make believe world, so that they magnify incidents which happen to them or invent them completely' (Heydon 1984).

There is a strong belief in legal circles that children are unreliable as witnesses due to their inability to understand what is real and what is unreal. This has led to cases of abuse against young children being dismissed in the courts as the children are regarded as being incompetent to testify. However, children's fantasies and play are based on what they know and have experienced.

> The cognitive and imaginative capabilities of three-year-olds do not enable them to describe anal intercourse and spitting out ejaculate for instance. Such detailed description from small children, in the absence of other factors, should be seen as stemming from the reality of past abuse rather than from their imagination. (Vizard et al 1987: p.24)

Another characteristic of young children's thinking is their belief that their thoughts and wishes have the power to alter the real world *(Magical Thinking)*. Children imbue adults with this magical power believing that they are all powerful and always right. They implicitly believe what an adult tells them with the consequence that threats can cause tremendous and long lasting fears.

> Jonathan was four years old when he accompanied his parents to the graveyard to place flowers on his grandmother's grave. He soon became bored and began jumping on the gravestones nearby. He ignored his parents when they told him to stop, but was terrified when they said 'If you jump on the gravestone the dead person will jump out of the grave and grab you!' To this day, Jonathan, now eleven years old, is terrified of graveyards and nothing can induce him to go near one.

It should not surprise us that fears are particularly common in the preschool child as the world must seem a bewildering place. Children in this age group typically fear ghosts and monsters but they do not falsely report sexual abuse as an exaggeration of a normal fear at any age. (Salter 1988: p.240)

When interviewing young children it must be remembered that cause and effect are only understood from a self-centred viewpoint. If two events occur together, they are deemed to be connected, as illustrated by the child who says ' I bumped my head because it was my birthday'. As a result young children may feel they have caused actions which occurred coincidentally.

> James (four years old) had been told off by his parents for getting his new clothes dirty when he was playing in the garden. Having been sent to bed he overheard his parents quarrelling downstairs. The next morning at breakfast his mother told him that daddy had gone away and wasn't going to be living with them anymore. James was quite convinced that daddy had left because he had been a naughty boy!

Young children are not able to concentrate on a task for very long and they commonly flit from one activity to another. Their attention is influenced by their interest in the material and as a result, most children's toys and books are colourfully designed. Long interviews are not appropriate at this age and the child's need to move around and engage in a variety of activities should be taken into account when planning a session.

Memory

Memory is an important cognitive skill which develops in tune with other aspects of the young child's development. Parents are often astonished at their young child's ability to remember events in the past which they may have forgotten, but what children remember depends on what they regard as significant and has meaning for them.

Young children are fairly good at recognising familiar stimuli, especially of the visual kind, but recall memory is much harder. For preschool children, part of their difficulty lies in the fact that they do not classify items for memory storage. Like adults, they are able to remember familiar and central events better than peripheral details. Children as young as two, three and four years have an ability to observe an incident in an almost photographic manner due to the fact that their observations are not affected by interpretation for meaning. Older children and adults on the other hand, try to make sense of what they see, and this may lead to inaccuracies in their recall. An adult who is questioning a child can often bring doubt into the child's mind by bringing meaning to the incident. The adult, as the all powerful being

who is always right, can cause children to doubt or change their statement. It is possible for a child (through fear or belief that the adult
knows best) to admit to wrong doing when questioned by an adult
when, in fact, they are innocent. In a study of early memories of
trauma, Terr (1988) found that: '$2^{1}/_{2}$ to 3 years appears to be about the
time most children will be able to lay down and later retrieve some sort
of verbal memory of trauma'. Some of the children in her study had
little or no verbal memories of what had happened to them but they
were able to show by means of their behaviour and play what had
occurred. Terr (1988) also noted that:

> verbal memories in children traumatised after $2^{1}/_{2}$ to 3 years will be fullest
> and closest to the accompanying documentation when the precipitating
> event is simple, short and surprising. Repeated and/or variable events (as
> in child abuse) are less fully remembered than are single episodes of
> trauma.

The reliability of children's memories has been a controversial topic
in establishing the credibility of the evidence in child sexual abuse
cases, and there has been a tendency to doubt the capacity of younger
children to recall events reliably. However, the inaccuracy of young
children's memory is not supported by the evidence, although it is true
that the amount they recall is often less. Fundudis (1989) makes the
point that 'for younger children, reference to context involving
familiarity based on regularity and routine (e.g bedtime, mealtime) is
even more important if they are to be expected to cope reliably with
recall'. It would appear that young children are more likely to miss
things out in their recall of an event rather than put things in which did
not happen. Young children can be facilitated in their recall by the use
of open-ended questions which leave them free to report the details
which are personally relevant to them. More specific questioning can
be used at a later stage to deal with any apparent inconsistencies.

Language in the preschool child

We cannot consider the young child's thinking without looking at how
language is acquired. In the preschool years, language develops at a
considerable rate and goes hand in hand with other aspects of the
child's development.

Between the ages of two and six years, children increase their
vocabulary to an average of between 8,000 and 14,000 words (Templin
1957) and master the basic grammatical rules of their native language.
Children in different language communities around the world appear
to go through the same stages in their acquisition of language skills.
When toddlers first start to put words together in early sentences they

use the important words to convey meaning (rather like a telegram) and miss out words such as 'the', 'to' and 'an'. However, their use of adult word order shows that they have a rudimentary knowledge of grammar and they can invent sentences they have never heard before e.g. 'Kitty comed home'. If children live in a rich language environment, this is clearly beneficial to their acquisition of sound language skills.

Understanding of language

We tend to regard understanding of language as preceding the ability to express it, but this is not as straightforward as it may seem. Children can often use language in seemingly appropriate contexts without a complete understanding of the concepts they are using. This often misleads adults into believing that children understand when they do not. When children attempt to interpret what we say to them, their interpretation is influenced by their knowledge of the words we use, and the context in which they are used. As adults, we must constantly check whether the words we use are in the child's vocabulary, and if so, whether they understand these words in the context in which we are using them. An excellent example of the kind of misunderstanding which can arise is to be found in Laurie Lee's account of his first day at school, quoted by M. Donaldson (Children's Minds):

> 'I spent the first day picking holes in paper then went home in a smouldering temper'.
> 'What's the matter love? Didn't he like it at school then?'
> 'They never gave me the present'.
> 'Present, what present?'
> 'They said they'd give me a present'.
> 'Well now, I'm sure they didn't'.
> 'They did! They said; 'You're Laurie Lee, aren't you? Well you just sit there for the present'.
> 'I sat there all day but I never got it. I ain't going back there again'.

Laurie clearly knew the word 'present', but not in the context in which the teacher used it. As adults it is all too easy for us to forget the gap between us and young children, and to believe we are communicating in a clear manner when in fact we are not. This may explain the reason why the answers young children often give to adults' questions are not necessarily appropriate to the questions asked.

The words to describe many sexual activities are not in the vocabulary of preschool children, and they have to explain what happened to them in terms of their own words and experience. Jan Hindman in *Just Before Dawn*: p.203, gives a good example of this:

In the interview of four-year-old Samuel, efforts are made to ascertain whether he is able to describe an erection or ejaculation. Samuel is asked 'What was his peepee doing?' Samuel replies, 'Oh it was sitting right up, big and wide awake', 'and what happened?', asked the examiner, 'I just kept touching it and touching it and touching it and touching it, up and down, up and down!', 'and then what happened?' asked the purple faced examiner, 'it just blew up!' said Samuel.

Some perpetrators appear to be aware of the child's limited vocabulary and give names to their activities such as 'the tickling game', which serves the purpose of protecting them should the child inform an adult. When Tina complains that she doesn't like 'the tickling game' the baby-sitter plays with her, it is essential for the adult to question Tina further, and not assume that tickling in this context is what we understand by the term.

As children at this stage in their development think in a literal manner and are unable to generalise, our questions should take this into account. Jan Hindman (1989: p.203) tells of the child who was being questioned as to whether or not her father had sexually touched her:

On the way home her mother asked her 'and daddy didn't ever touch you in your private parts?', 'No' says Mandy, and after taking another lick of her popsicle, Mandy flatly stated to her mother 'but daddy lets me suck on his Weiner all the time!'

Lack of logical sequencing

Preschool children do not logically organise their thinking or speech as the young child cannot recall information sequentially. Instead, they say whatever enters their mind at the moment, without much censoring or prethought, and their narratives tend to be disjointed and rambling. They recount an incident from their own viewpoint and often assume that the adult has the same knowledge of the situation as they do. Young children are unable to put themselves in the place of another person (egocentrism) and therefore do not understand what the adult knows or doesn't know, and what they need to be told. When young children are giving an account of their abuse, it can often be difficult for the adult to get a clear picture of what has happened due to this inability to sequence.

Concepts

The concepts of time, number and distance are poorly understood by preschool children even when they may be able to use the words associated with these concepts. The adult, therefore, has to check what the child's understanding is, by phrasing questions containing these concepts in various ways. Young children have great difficulty in understanding what time is, and how long it will take for something to happen. Any adult who has made a long car journey with young children will understand the difficulty of explaining how long the journey will take, and will be faced with frequent demands to know 'Are we there yet?'

As with other concepts, time has to be attached to something meaningful to the child and within the child's own experience. Techniques such as talking about the number of sleeps, or making marks on a calendar have to be used to assist the child's understanding. Young children can only tell 'when' something happened if it can be associated with a significant event in their normal routine.

When preschool children are interviewed about sexual abuse, they are often asked 'how often' an activity has occurred. This is an impossible question for them, but they will often feel obliged to answer in order to please the examiner. They may select a number at random or, through fear of blame, answer 'once'. Some young children are able to recite numbers in sequence, but we must not be fooled by this trick into believing that they understand the concept of number. Unless these limitations are understood by adults, the children's statements can often be seen as unreliable and doubt is cast on their truthfulness.

Personality and social development

As preschool children are changing physically and developing new skills, they are also acquiring views of themselves as persons. They are increasingly exposed to a lifelong process of socialisation as their horizons widen beyond the immediate family. The family is the primary social group and it is likely to provide the most powerful formative influence on the development of the child's personality. In the early years, children have to learn to trust others and develop a sense of who they are. If their early attachments have been poor, this affects their ability to make progress emotionally and socially, and they become anxious and insecure in the face of new experiences.

The development of a self-concept is a gradual one, but the beginnings are observable in the preschool years. At first children define themselves in terms of their physical appearance and what they do, but as they grow older, they use more psychological descriptions such as 'I am clever', 'I am a good boy'. Erikson (1963) theorised that children develop their personality by resolving various developmental crises at different stages in life. These crises focus on the conflicts between the child and the social environment which places demands and restrictions upon the child's behaviour. Infants have to learn that all their needs cannot be met instantaneously and the way mothers achieve this sets the platform for future development. Although preschool children are enthusiastic and full of initiative, they have to learn to attend to the wishes of others.

How does this learning come about? Having formed a strong bond to certain individuals, children will inevitably wish to conform to their standards of behaviour. They do this by identifying with them and incorporating their ways of behaving. The little boy wants to be 'like daddy' and the little girl 'like mummy'. From an early age boys and girls are expected to behave differently and by the time they are three years old, they have formed definite sex appropriate preferences with regard to toys which tend to strengthen with age. To some extent, this is due to direct training by parents, but there is evidence which suggests that it is also a result of identification with the same sex parent. In a study of five-year-old boys, Mussen and Distler (1959) found that boys with a high male identification tended to see their fathers as warmer and more affectionate than boys with low male identification. The same results were found for girls' identification with their mothers. It would appear that it is the positive rather than the negative qualities of parents which encourage identification.

As children have more contact with the outside world, other influences come to bear on the way they view themselves. Mixing with other children in the playgroup or nursery teaches children about taking turns, sharing and attending to the needs of others. Inevitably problems arise, and there can sometimes be outbursts of aggressive behaviour over the possession of toys or the control of space. As aggression is regarded as a male trait, it is often fostered in boys by contact with their fathers. At this age, children readily imitate aggression displayed by adults or shown on television. When something is troubling young children we are most likely to see this reflected in the way they behave due to their limited cognitive and language skills.

The sexual abuse of very young children has become increasingly recognised and several surveys have found that one third or more of their victim samples are under the age of six years (Gale et al 1988). There is a continuing debate over the short and long term effects of sexual abuse in the preschool child although this is an area where there is a dearth of experimental investigation. Some researchers argue that because the young child has little or no understanding of the sexual nature of the experience, the emotional trauma is less enduring. Others argue that preschool children are especially vulnerable because they are in the early stages of psychosexual development and the long term effects are therefore more damaging. Although some young children are symptom free at disclosure, others show marked symptoms, mainly of a somatic or behavioural nature. In a report by Mian et al (1986) which focused exclusively on 125 abused children six years of age and under, it was found that two thirds showed behavioural and/or physical symptoms.

Many symptoms of sexual abuse have been identified in young children and the following table lists those most commonly found. (*Sexual Abuse of Young Children*, MacFarlane, Waterman et al 1986: p114.)

Type of effect	Specific problem noted
Affective effects	Anxiety; depression; anger.
Physical effects	Injury, bruises and/or bleeding in external genitalia, vagina, anus; problems walking or sitting; sexually transmitted diseases.
Psychosomatic effects	Stomachaches; headaches; encopresis; enuresis; sleep disturbance.
Cognitive problems	Hypothesised (e.g. problems with concentration).
Behavioural problems	Acting out; withdrawal; regression; repetition with other children and toys such as dolls.
Psychopathology	Manifested in various ways; present in a significant number of cases.
Sexuality	Excessive masturbation; repetition of sexual acts with others; atypical sexual knowledge; concerns and preoccupation with sexual matters.
Interpersonal problems	Withdrawal; avoidance; occasionally over-familiarity.

Many of these symptoms, of course, may be found in children of all ages, but in the younger child, behaviour disturbance or injury is more likely to be the presenting symptom. Physical effects are much less frequently reported but they do occur in some children. Venereal infection of the mouth, anus or vagina and compulsive masturbation are common symptoms found in the under fives (Vizard and Tranter 1988). Frozen watchfulness and anxious attachment can also be observed in some sexually abused young children, and this may link to the finding that at least 15 per cent of sexually abused children have also been physically abused.

Due to the multiplicity of symptoms observed in the young sexually abused child, many of which have valid alternative explanations, their usefulness as behavioural indicators has been questioned. Gale et al (1988), in a study of sexual abuse in young children found that inappropriate sexual behaviour was the symptom which distinguished the group of sexually abused children from groups of physically abused or non-abused children. If this is indeed the case, then it is essential that we are aware of what constitutes normal sexual behaviour in the under fives.

Sexual development

Very little has been written about the sexual development of young children and society likes to think of this group as sexually innocent. However, Freud's theories of the oral and anal stage of psychosexual development drew attention to the fact that young children do have sexual feelings. Genital play and masturbation are quite common and preschool children have a fascination about bodily functions. Young children are also interested in examining the bodies of other children of a similar age. These are all developmentally appropriate behaviours, but when a child masturbates in a compulsive manner, preferring this activity to play with other children, there is cause for concern. The sexually abused child may involve toys or objects in the masturbation activity and attempt to insert these in the vagina or rectum. Non-abused children do not typically use force to engage another child in sexual activity or simulate copulation with a toy or another child. Evidence of sexual activity or knowledge which is not age appropriate should always be regarded as requiring further investigation.

How does the young child decide what is good or bad?

In the field of moral development Piaget and Kohlberg have been the most influential figures in enabling us to understand how moral judgement develops. Piaget (1932) maintained that children below the ages of three or four years are 'premoral' in that they do not understand rules and so do not make judgements. From the ages of three to six years, children see rules as absolute and unchangeable. If a rule is broken then punishment is inevitable and 'goodness' and 'badness' are judged on the consequences rather than the intent. Children at this stage would view five glasses being broken accidentally as more naughty than one glass broken intentionally. However, Nelson (1980) found that children of three or four years of age can be aware of intention or motive and will take it into account if it is made clear and salient.
    Most of the studies by Kohlberg and Piaget posed dilemmas

concerned with wrongdoing for children to deal with, but this does not tell us anything about the kind of reasoning children use to justify good behaviour. Eisenberg and her colleagues (1986) explored these questions and found that the preschool child is concerned with a self-centred orientation, i.e. what feels good to me is right. This, of course, is what one would expect when one remembers the egocentric nature of the young child's thinking.

Clearly the young child has very limited notions of what is right or wrong and cannot make judgements about an activity such as sexual abuse. If the activity gives pleasure and satisfies other basic needs they may well cooperate with the sexual act and experience no feelings of guilt. On the other hand, some children as young as four years seem aware of the inappropriateness of such activities and are relieved when they do not have to 'play those dirty games anymore'.

The young child's concept of illness

When trying to understand illness or death, the young child brings to this task the same limitations we have observed in all other areas of their development. Several studies have shown that children have some startling misapprehensions about the reasons why people become ill. In interviews with children hospitalised for heart disease and diabetes, 90 per cent answered the question 'Why do children get sick?' with the response, 'because they are bad' (Beverley 1936). Some children see illness as a punishment, and having to be admitted to hospital as a sign of rejection by their parents. Fortunately hospitals are now more aware of the child's feelings and allow parents, especially those of young children, to stay in hospital with their child. Children (like adults) are afraid of medical procedures, especially if needles are involved, and this may compound their ideas of being punished. When children have frequent periods of illness or hospitalisation, this can have a detrimental effect on their general development

For the young child who is found to be HIV positive, other negative connotations come into play. Due to fear and uninformed attitudes towards people with AIDS, children and their families may be socially isolated and the children deprived of the opportunity to mix with others and take part in fun activities. Other seriously ill children, such as those suffering from cancer or heart disease, receive a great deal of sympathy from the public and often money is raised to provide them with treats. Children who are HIV positive are not regarded in the same way however, and their illness is surrounded with secrecy and shame. When children have an illness it is important to check with them why they think they are ill, and to give information at a suitable developmental level to ensure they do not blame themselves.

Summary

- Preschool children do not reason in a logical manner as they view the world from their own perspective. The adult must attempt to get to the child's level and accommodate to the limitations of the child.

- Young children have a limited understanding of causality and concepts of time and number. They regard adults as being all powerful and having superior knowledge and can be unduly influenced by these factors in the interview setting.

- Although young children can recall fewer details than older children, what they do remember tends to be accurate. What is remembered is what has personal significance for the child, and they have difficulty selecting relevant from irrelevant features.

- Communication with the preschool child has to use age appropriate language and it is essential that the adult checks the child's understanding of what has been said. They are unable to relate an incident in a chronological or logical manner and cannot assess what the adult already knows and what they need to know.

- Although young children can confuse what is real and unreal, their fantasies are based on what they know and have experienced. They are not able to fantasise about sexual abuse or to give explicit sexual information except through direct experiences. Due to their limited cognitive and verbal skills, young children usually indicate what has happened to them by means of their play and behaviour.

- The concept of illness is poorly understood and young children may feel they are to blame and are being punished when they have to undergo medical procedures. Being HIV positive can isolate the preschool child and deny them interaction with their peer group.

References

Beverley B, 1936 The effects of illness upon emotional development. *Journal of Paediatrics* **8** (553).

Donaldson M, 1978 *Children's minds.* Fontana.

Eisenberg N, 1986 *Altruistic emotion, cognition and behaviour.* N J Erlbaum, Hillsdale.

Erikson E H, 1963 *Childhood and society* 2nd edn. Norton, New York.

Flavell J H, 1963 *The developmental psychology of Jean Piaget.* Van Nostrand, Princeton, New Jersey.

Fundudis T, 1989 Children's memory and the assessment of possible child sex abuse. *Journal of Child Psychology and Psychiatry* **30** (3): 337–46.

Gale J, Thompson R J, Moran T, Sack W H, 1988 Sexual Abuse in Young Children: its clinical presentation and characteristic patterns. *Child Abuse and Neglect* **12**: 163–70.

Heydon J, 1984 *Evidence cases and materials.* 2nd edn. Butterworths.

Hindman J, 1989 *Just before dawn.* Alexandria Associates, Oregon.

King M A and Yuille J C, 1987 Suggestibility and the child witness. In Ceci S J, Toglia M P and Ross A F (eds) *Childrens eyewitness memory.* Springer, New York.

MacFarlane K, Waterman J, Conerly S, Damon L, Durfee M, Long S, 1986 *Sexual abuse of young children.* Guilford Press, New York.

Mian M, Wehrspann W, Klajner-Diamond H, Le Baron D, Winder C, 1986 Review of 125 children 6 years of age and under who were sexually abused. *Child Abuse and Neglect* **10**: 223–29.

Mussen P and Distler L, 1959 Masculinity, identification and father-son relationships. *Journal Abnormal Social Psychology,* **59**: 350–56

Nelson S A, 1980 Factors influencing young children's use of motives and outcomes as moral criteria. *Child Development* **51**: 823–29.

Piaget J, 1929 *The childs' conception of the world.* Harcourt and Brace, New York.

Piaget J, 1932 *The moral judgement of the child.* Macmillan, New York.

Piaget J, 1954 *The construction of reality in the child.* Basic Books, New York.

Salter A C, 1988 *Treating child sex offenders and victims.* Sage, California.

Templin M C, 1957 *Certain language skills in children: their development and interrelationships.* University of Minnesota Institute of Child Welfare Monograph 26.

Terr L, 1988 Case study. What happens to early memories of trauma? A study of twenty children under age five at the time of documented traumatic events. *J Am Acad Child Adolesc Psychiatry* 1988 **27** (1): 96–103.

Vizard E, Bentovim A, Tranter M, 1987 Interviewing sexually abused children. *Adoption and Fostering* **11**: 20–27.

Vizard E, Tranter M, 1988 Recognition and assessment of child sexual abuse. In Bentovin A, Elton A, Hildegrand J, Tranter M, Vizard E (eds) *Child sexual abuse within the family, assessment and treatment.* John Wright.

2 School age children (5-11 years)

Introduction

When children enter full time education around the age of five years they face new challenges and expectations. In any reception class you will find children with a wide variety of skills and at different levels of development. Some are eager and ready to meet the new experiences, while others are fearful and unsure and may be operating at a level typical of a younger child. Those who have had experience of nursery education have been introduced to many of the skills they will use in the classroom. For others this will be their first experience of separation from mother, and it may take some time for them to adjust. In the primary school, children build on their achievements of the preschool years and acquire new intellectual skills. They spend an increasing amount of time outside the home, at school and with their friends, and their dependency on their parents decreases as they are exposed to these new influences.

Cognitive skills

In the first two years of schooling there are still limitations on the child's thought processes and many of the characteristics of the preschool child's thinking are still evident. Many five and six year olds are still egocentric in their thinking and have a limited grasp of many concepts. However, around the age of six or seven a remarkable shift occurs in their ability to understand, and they begin to think in a more logical and rational manner. Piaget labelled this stage of development 'concrete operational thought' as children are able to manipulate symbols logically but their thinking is still heavily reliant on their own experiences. At the infant school stage, for example, children rely on concrete objects such as bricks when they are learning to count and they have to establish what is known as 'one to one correspondence' that is each number corresponds to an object. It is also easier for them to understand if the objects are familiar to them, e.g. the question $2+2 =?$ is more difficult when put in this abstract form than if expressed, 'if I had two sweets and you gave me two more sweets, how many sweets would I have then? Children have to reason from the particular to the abstract and not *vice versa*. At school, children are faced with having to learn new skills such as decoding print, dealing with number concepts, and controlling a pencil in order to reproduce symbols on a page. They have to understand that the printed word stands for the words we use when we speak, and in the early stages of this process, children will often confuse letters and number symbols. Adults begin to make assessments of what the child can and cannot do, and formal learning becomes of prime importance.

As the concept of number begins to have meaning for them they are able to deal with abstract manipulations such as addition, subtraction, multiplication and division. However, when a sexually abused child is questioned as to the frequency of abuse, they are often unable to give an accurate account. This may be due to the fact that the abuse has occurred on a regular basis over a long period of time, and adults in the same situation would be equally unable to respond in a meaningful manner. 'Lots of times' or a 'few times' are more realistic measures for a child, and it is not appropriate that they should be pressured to give a more exact calculation.

Concept of time

The school aged child gradually learns about measuring time, by learning to tell what time it is on a clock, but they still have great difficulty in understanding intervals of time. When asked to estimate how long an activity took, they frequently overestimate. Large intervals of time such as a month or a year mean very little to them, and this explains the problems they face when trying to understand the time scale of historical events. For time to have meaning for the child it must be attached to significant events in their own experience such as birthdays, Christmas, school holidays etc. It is essential for the adult to understand these limitations and to question the child, with regard to the timing of events, in a manner which facilitates them pinpointing an event in conjunction with events which have significance for them. It may be possible for children to give an accurate timing of when an event occurred if they can use reference points such as a football match, attending a club, or going swimming. The question of timing is often a crucial factor in a child's verbal account of abuse as adults will often attempt to dismiss the credibility of the child's statement by providing evidence that they were elsewhere when the child claimed the abuse occurred. Children are not able to give accurate estimates of time unless the incident can be associated with their usual routine.

Many researchers have listed school failure as one of the symptoms observable in children of this age range who have been sexually abused. As these children are commonly found to be either withdrawn, depressed, and removed from school interests and activities, or angry, aggressive and disruptive, it is clear that school performance is likely to be affected. Sexually abused children are under stress, and their ability to attend to what is happening in the classroom, and to absorb new experiences is likely to be impaired. They accordingly fall behind with their school work and their problems are compounded. The case of Donna illustrates this point:

> Donna was severely abused at home from an early age and she performed poorly in school despite being of average ability. She was unable to concentrate on her school work as she was preoccupied with the dread of having to return home. As the school day progressed she became increasingly anxious and would often volunteer to stay behind and clear up, simply to postpone the inevitable return home and resumption of abuse. On one occasion, the class was given the task of writing a story about what they were thinking. Donna was unable to put pencil to paper, such was her dread of giving away any information which would betray her abuse and get her into further trouble at home.

On the other hand, some abused children find school a haven, arriving early and staying late. They appear to be able to involve themselves in their work to such a degree that they can shut out all other thoughts at least for that part of the day.

Memory

By the time children are seven years old their capacity to remember improves significantly, mainly because they begin to use strategies which assist in recall. They learn to classify objects, and one of the most frequent pastimes of this group is collecting things and arranging them in relation to each other. This skill of classification develops over the primary school years as Neimark (1971) demonstrated in an experiment. Children aged between six and twelve years were shown pictures relating to four categories — animals, furniture, clothing and transportation. Without telling them that all the pictures belonged to these categories, the children were asked to arrange the pictures in any way which would help them to remember. The younger children, aged six to eight years old, for the most part made no effort to classify the pictures. However, older children made increasingly harder efforts to do so. The more proficient they were in this, the better they recalled the pictures at a later time. Other techniques such as breaking down lists into smaller groups (e.g. telephone numbers) and making a sentence of an otherwise meaningless sequence, (e.g. Every Good Boy Deserves Favours) are commonly acquired. Attempting to assess the differences in memory capacity according to age by laboratory techniques has fallen out of fashion in recent years, and researchers are now using more realistic situations to try and assess how well a child remembers events.

> These experiments show that children's memories can be very powerful and that age difference in memory performance can easily be reversed. For example, if children have superior knowledge of the subject matter (eg chess or prehistoric monsters), they can remember more information than adults in a standard memory test (Chi and Ceci 1986).

The same would be true of an eyewitnessing situation where, for example, 'a child who has a detailed knowledge of cars is likely to give a better vehicle description than the average adult'. (Spencer and Flin: p.239). What is clear from the research is that children tend to pay more attention to events and details that have personal significance for them and these may not be the same as for adults.

In the field of child sexual abuse, the accuracy of children's memories has been a controversial topic and doubt has often been cast on their ability to give accurate accounts of events which happened in the past, especially if the events are of a traumatic nature. However, modern psychological and medical research suggests that children are much more reliable as witnesses than previously thought (Spencer and Flin: p.237). When children are asked to freely recall what has happened, the information has been found to be accurate in general, but the amount of information is reduced. When questioned in a specific manner, young children are found to be less accurate in their responses than older children. Young children have particular difficulty in reporting precise details of time, speed or distance and this matches what we know of the development of these concepts in the child. In many ways, the limitations of the child's memory are similar to those of adults, as it is easier to remember what actually happened than the descriptive information. By the time a case comes to court, there is usually a long time delay between the abusive incident and having to give evidence about it. Dent and Stephenson (1972) tested 10 and 11 year old children's memory of a film of a theft and found that after a delay of up to two months, the accuracy of the information was maintained, but the overall amount of information recalled was diminished. It would appear then, that children's memories are no less accurate than those of adults, but they do differ in the amount of information they are able to recall.

It has also been commonly held that children '...because of their immaturity are very suggestible and can easily be influenced both by adults and other children' (Heydon 1984). It is true that children are anxious to please adults and tend to view them as having superior knowledge and therefore being infallible must be right. However, when Gail Goodman studied whether children were easily led when questioned about personally significant events such as sexual abuse, she found that children as young as four years were remarkably resistant to suggestive questions. In a court setting, children are often exposed to repeated questioning when they are being cross examined and Moston (1987) found that this reduced the number of correct responses in children aged 6 to 10 years. He hypothesises that this may partially explain why children appear to be suggestible as they can become confused and contradict themselves. The child's own account of the abuse is frequently the main, or sole, evidence against a perpetrator and the reliability of children's evidence depends so crucially on how they are questioned. It is important that they are interviewed as soon as possible in a manner which facilitates their recall.

Language

As children progress through the primary school their ability to handle language increases and they can recognise that words can have more than one meaning. This is illustrated in the child's humour at this stage when they become able to play with words and are fascinated by puns e.g. the many variations of the knock, knock jokes. They are increasingly able to consider several ideas at the same time, and they are not tied to their own perspective of the world. Language complexity develops with the child's growing cognitive skills and they can increasingly recount events in a logical sequence which makes their communications more easily understood by adults. The school aged child's verbal account of abuse has increased detail, precision and clarity although they still do not have an understanding of adult sexual language and have to use their own words to describe what happened.

Special needs children

Children with special needs pose particular problems as their development of language and cognitive skills may be at a level considerably lower than their chronological age. Those with severe and complex problems are usually identified in the preschool years and receive specialised provision. However, integration of children with special needs into mainstream education is increasingly common as a result of the *Education Act 1981*, and adults interviewing children should be aware of this. In dealing with many of these children, specialist advice will be essential as the normal methods of communication may not be appropriate, as in cases of hearing or visually impaired children.

Although there has been a lack of research into the links between child sexual abuse and learning difficulties, there are pointers that these children may be particularly vulnerable due to their limited understanding and high dependency on adults. Like the preschool child, they can be taken advantage of more readily, and with limited verbal skills they often have to communicate that something is troubling them by means of their behaviour. However, problem behaviour is too often seen as the normal pattern for many of these children and is linked to their disability. Symptoms which may signal alarm in a child without a handicap are not seen as possible indicators of abuse. Children with a physical or mental handicap have reduced independence from adults and appropriate body boundaries are not able to be established, placing them at greater risk.

Social and emotional development

As children become less egocentric in the concrete stage of operational thinking, they are able to understand how others perceive situations. The impact of friends, relatives and teachers has increasing significance as they receive negative and positive messages about the kind of person they are. Erikson described this stage of personality development as 'industry versus inferiority', and children develop views of themselves as 'workers'. This is the age when children of all cultures receive instruction in the ways of the world, and in our culture most of this is formalised in the school curriculum. It is the stage, therefore, when competence is acquired in both cognitive and social skills, but not all children are equally successful in demonstrating their competence and many experience failure. Consequently, they form a view of themselves as inadequate or inferior and believe they cannot succeed. This can build into a vicious circle when the discouraged child refuses to tackle tasks, believing their failure is inevitable. Becoming more aware of others and their achievements causes children to alter their perception of themselves and they use the personal characteristics of others as standards to evaluate themselves (Rholes and Ruble 1984). Their descriptions of themselves become less global and more specific, that is not simply 'good' or 'bad', but 'good at drawing but not so good at reading'. By the age of 9 or 10 years, children are very self-critical and, as a result, particularly sensitive to correction and embarrassment. Having a good feeling about oneself is important for all areas of development and Coopersmith (1967) found that children with high self-esteem were more independent and creative, did better in school, were more likely to be assertive, socially outgoing and popular with their peers.

Many researchers have listed poor self-esteem as one of the long term effects of child sexual abuse. Smith (1992) states that 'a child who has been sexually abused for as long as they can remember may fail to even establish a sense of themselves… Some children who have been sexually abused perceive their self worth only in terms of their sexuality. They feel valued only as a sexual object and relate to the world through sexual activity sometimes exclusively. It is not uncommon for children who have been sexually abused to feel insignificant, worthless and almost invisible'. When children's feelings about themselves are so severely damaged they feel unable to compete with their peer groups and fail to acknowledge any successes they may achieve.

For the primary school child, the peer group begins to assume a greater importance in their lives and stable relationships, usually with children of the same gender, are established. Friendships are important for the growth of the child's social self and as well as providing companionship, the peer group can be a useful testing ground for trying out new behaviours and gaining knowledge. By the age of five or six years, children have developed gender constancy, that is they know that you don't change gender by changing your appearance. This is also the time when ideas about the differing sex roles are more rigidly applied. Girls, however, would appear to have less stereotyped concepts and often indulge in behaviour which is regarded as being boyish, although the reverse is not true. Perhaps girls are aware, even at this age, that male attributes are more valued in society.

Children learn the rules they have to obey if they are to gain acceptance by their peers and breaking these rules can have serious consequences. Parents are only too aware of the influence of other children's behaviour on their own child and are often anxious if they associate with children whose behaviour they find undesirable. If children do not learn how to get on with others, they are rejected by the groups and become socially isolated, or resort to playing with much younger children. Reacting to rejection by aggressive outbursts and attention seeking behaviour simply reinforces isolation from the peer group. It is often very difficult to break this pattern and enable the child to become more socially acceptable, and those who are rejected or unpopular tend to remain so throughout their childhood. The seriousness of failing to develop socially acceptable behaviour is highlighted by Hartup (1984) who found that 'rejection by one's peers in elementary school is one of the very few aspects of childhood functioning that consistently predicts behaviour problems or emotional disturbances in adolescence and adulthood'.

It is not uncommon for children who have been sexually abused to show behavioural difficulties such as aggression or withdrawal from social contact. These behaviours, as we have seen, may cause them to be disliked or rejected by other children, thus compounding their poor image of themselves. Through communication with their peers, sexually abused children learn that their experiences are not typical, and they can have a growing awareness of their difference from others and the need to keep their experiences secret. Moreover, overt sexualised behaviour can meet with censure from the peer group as children become increasingly aware that this behaviour is not socially acceptable.

Moral development

In the early years of the primary school, children still view rules as absolute and unchangeable, but gradually as they develop the ability to see the other person's viewpoint, they are able to take into account the other person's needs even if these conflict with their own needs. Children in this age group see punishment as a natural consequence of breaking rules and are much more severe than adults in the punishments they deem as appropriate for bad behaviour. By the time they reach the age of ten there is an understanding that rules can be changed and children make up their own rules by agreement as they play games. Actions by this stage are judged more by the intention than the consequences, and the child who broke the glass on purpose would be regarded as naughtier than the one who accidentally broke five glasses. Children also see the necessity for making amends for doing wrong and will suggest ways of expressing contrition. We must of course remember that although children (like adults) understand and accept moral standards, they do not necessarily act on them. There is often a difference between what one knows is right and what one actually does.

Some abused children are given confusing messages about what is right and wrong by the perpetrator, especially if the abuse occurs within a caring relationship. Children are often trapped into compliance because of a desire to please the adult, especially if that adult has many positive qualities. In attempting to make sense of a situation, the child may reason that 'as daddy is good, he wouldn't do a bad thing', and he may also have told her that 'daddy is doing this because he loves you so much'. Having special treats and privileges as a result of the abuse can trick a child into believing that the behaviour is not wrong. As we first learn what is right and wrong from our parents, the abusing parent can often convince the child that what is happening is acceptable. Sexually abused children become increasingly aware that what they have been doing is seen as bad by others in society, and they can develop strong feelings of guilt and self-blame. They see themselves as deserving of punishment and this is often reinforced by threats from the perpetrator. However, we must constantly bear in mind that not all children react to sexual abuse in a similar manner, and there is a wide variation ranging from apparent lack of symptoms to serious disturbance. Gomez-Schwartz, et al (1990) found that 'the failure to acquire socially valued behaviours (prosocial deficit), a characteristic of the younger children was not an issue for many of the school-age youngsters'.

Sexual development

Freud described this stage of psychosexual development as the latency period believing that the early sexual impulses of the young child decreased and were not reawakened until puberty. However, subsequent research has demonstrated that the latency period is largely a myth and the interest in sexual matters continues through the middle childhood years. The sexualised games involving exploration and touching are still indulged in, but as adult disapproval becomes more apparent, such games are more likely to be secretive in nature. Even during the period when friendships are mainly same sex, there still appears to be considerable heterosexual interest and some age appropriate sexual activity. One survey found that the majority of 10 to 12 year old children claim to have had a special friend of the opposite sex and at 10 years, two thirds claimed to have kissed this girl/boy friend. Masturbation tends to increase in frequency and boys of this age are likely to be engaged in games such as seeing who can 'piss' the furthest or highest. Jokes progress from the typical 'lavatorial' jokes of the younger children to more sexual ones, and sexual words can be used to shock even if their understanding of the meaning is unsure.

Jan Hindman referred to the sexually abused victim at this stage of development as being 'the unfortunate'. As children become aware of the significance of sexuality she explains that the abused child is 'constantly looking back to a stage in development when they were cooperative, acquiescent or, at a minimum, unable to stop the abuse... They are constantly looking back, criticising themselves and stumbling at attempts to go forward'. As the child approaches puberty they learn about reproduction and may become aware for the first time of what is happening to them in the abusive situation. Sex education programmes are increasingly used in schools and children hear sexual words that relate to their own abusive experience. However, most do not react with anger towards the perpetrator, but rather with disgust towards themselves for what they did. We can assume then that increasing sexual awareness for the abused child can indeed be unfortunate as it is associated with negative feelings of disgust and shame directed towards themselves.

School child and illness

With the growth of cognitive skills, children between the ages of five and 11 are increasingly able to understand illness in more logical and abstract terms as compared to the magical thinking of the preschool child. By the time children are about seven years old they understand the idea of germs causing illness but they have rather odd notions of how they operate inside the body. 'When you get a cold...bacteria get in by breathing...then the lungs get too soft and it goes to the nose' (Gross p.79).

Gellert, in a study of children's beliefs about illness, found that two thirds of children aged four to 16 (both healthy and hospitalised) blamed themselves to some extent for an illness, feeling that it followed doing something you shouldn't do or not doing something you should. Even as adults it is easy to return to the magical thinking stage when our emotions are involved, as can be seen from many people's attitudes towards those who have AIDS. When we are fearful and lack accurate information about an illness such as AIDS, it is all too easy for our ability to feel pity for the victims to be inhibited, and we are more likely to make insensitive comments.

Living with a life threatening disease causes enormous stress in children and their families and we need to help children with this stress in an age appropriate manner. Allen and Green have made a useful contribution in this area by adapting material for use with children.

Children's inability to understand the gravity of their illness is a reason often put forward by parents for saying very little to them, but this may be saying more about the feelings of the parents than those of the child. Work with dying children has shown that they wish to be involved in discussions and decisions about their health and they are often more realistic about outcomes than their parents. The false optimism of parents can place a great strain on the child, and adults and children can enter a mutual pretence that death is not imminent (Bluebond-Langer). Of course we have to take into account the child's understanding of death and this changes as the child grows older. Around the age of seven, children appear to grasp the idea that death is inevitable and universal, but they still resist the idea that they have to die. As concrete thinkers, they are interested in detailed explanations such as what happens to your body when you die. When children are dying they need to have their fears and anxieties dealt with openly in an age appropriate manner. Unless they are actively encouraged to do this they may suppress these feelings in order to protect their parents.

Children who acquire a life threatening illness can look back to a time when they were once fit and healthy and the loss of their strength and control over their bodies can give rise to feelings of frustration and anger. To add to their problems they have to cope with an emotionally upset family who are no longer able to offer the same level of support due to their own distress. Some children respond by becoming withdrawn and regressing in their behaviour to a younger age, whereas others may indulge in aggressive and angry outbursts. Yet others may become unnaturally good and forbearing.

Children who are HIV positive need counselling not only about the nature of their illness, but also about how to cope with possible rejection and hostility from other children and adults. AIDS has entered the child's world and already we hear of children playing games when they call out to another child 'you've got AIDS'. As with sexual abuse, HIV infection is surrounded by secrecy and becomes associated with shame and prejudice. This could result in children losing friends, isolating themselves, and refusing (or being refused permission) to attend school.

Summary

- Children at the concrete operational stage become more logical and less egocentric in their thinking processes, but they are still reliant on their own experiences.

- Concepts of time and number are increasingly understood but must be related to the child's routine or significant events in order to provide any degree of accuracy.

- Children in this age group begin to use strategies which help them to remember. Recent research indicates that children can recall accurately and are less suggestible if questioned in an appropriate manner.

- Those children with special needs may be particularly vulnerable to abuse due to their limited understanding and high dependency on adults. The need for specialist help when dealing with these children is stressed.

- Sexual abuse can affect the intellectual, social and emotional development of a child, causing academic failure, social isolation and poor self-esteem.

- As children become more aware of the significance of sexuality, those who have been abused often experience negative feelings towards themselves and feel responsible for what happened to them.

- Children need to be involved in discussion about their illness and have an opportunity to express their fears and anxieties. For those children who become HIV positive, counselling is essential to enable them to cope with the additional burden of possible rejection and social isolation.

References

Allen D A, Green V P, 1988 Helping children cope with stress. *Early Child Development and Care* **37**: 1–11.

Bluebond-Langer M, 1978 *The private worlds of dying children.* Princeton University Press, US.

Chi M, Ceci S, 1986 Content knowledge and the reorganisation of memory. In Reese H W, Lipsitt L (eds) *Advances in child development and behaviour* **20**: 1–37.

Coopersmith S, 1967 *The antecedents of self-esteem.* Freeman, San Francisco.

Dent H R, Stephenson G M, 1979 Identification evidence: experimental investigations of factors affecting the reliability of juvenile and adult witnesses. In Farrington D, Hawkins K, Lloyd-Bostock S (eds) *Psychology, Law and Legal Processes.* Humanities Press, Atlantic Highlands NJ, US.

Gellert E, 1965 Children's beliefs about bodily illness, paper presented at 1965 meeting of the American Psychological Association, quoted in Perrin E C, Gerrity P S 'There's a Demon in Your Belly' *Paediatrics* **67**: 841–49.

Gomes-Schwartz B, Horowitz J M, Cardarelli A P, 1990 *Child sexual abuse, the initial effects.* Sage Publications, California, US.

Goodman G, Clark-Stewart A, 1990 Suggestibility in children's testimony: implications for child sexual abuse investigations. In Doris J (ed) *The suggestibility of children's recollections* American Psychological Association, Washington DC, US.

Gross J, 1989 *Psychology and parenthood.* Open University Press.

Hartup W W, 1984 The Peer Context in Middle Childhood. In Collins W A (ed) *Development during middle childhood. The years from six to twelve.* National Academy Press, Washington DC, US.

Heydon J, 1984 *Evidence cases and materials.* 2nd edn., Butterworths.

Hindman J, 1989 *Just before dawn.* Alexandria Associates, Oregon.

Moston S, 1987 The suggestibility of children in interview studies. *First Language* **7**: 67–78.

Neimark E D, Slotnick N, Ulrich T, 1971 Development of memorisation strategies. *Developmental psychology* **5**: 427-32.

Rholes W, Ruble D, 1984 Children's understanding of dispositional characteristics of others. *Child Development* **55**: 550–60.

Smith G, 1992 The unbearable traumatogenic past: child sexual abuse. In V. P. Varma (ed) *The secret life of vulnerable children.* Routledge, London

Spencer J R, Flin R, 1990 *The evidence of children.* Blackstone.

3 Adolescents

Introduction

The transitional period between childhood and adulthood which we refer to as adolescence is triggered by the changes which occur in the young person's body. Society has tended to see this stage of development as one of great stress and drama and we assume that all adolescents have to go through a difficult passage to arrive at adult status. Teenagers can be difficult to live with due to the fact that they are experiencing dramatic changes not only in their physical characteristics, but also in their social and emotional development. Many parents feel that they are living with a stranger, if not a monster, and both adolescents and their parents have to face major readjustments in their relationships with each other. However, some adolescents do manage to cope with these changes more easily than others, and if the young person has successfully negotiated the earlier stages of their development, then the adjustments to adolescence can be completed without undue drama.

Young people enter adolescence at different ages and there are early and late developers in both sexes. One only needs to look at the variation in size and shape in a class of children in the first year of secondary education for this to become apparent. Many more girls are experiencing their first menstruation while still in primary school and it would appear that girls in general are about two years ahead of boys in pubertal development. Those who develop early may well have an advantage but they are also faced with the greater expectations adults place on them by virtue of their more mature appearance.

Cognitive development

Piaget referred to this stage of cognitive development as 'formal operational thought'. The child is beginning to move from thinking tied to concrete operations to an ability to reason in the abstract and form hypotheses. Adolescents are increasingly able to operate on a level of theory and to think mentally about a problem before attempting a practical solution. The style of secondary education reflects this change and learning becomes more formal and theoretical in nature. Not all children achieve mastery of these cognitive skills at the same time, and many children with learning difficulties remain at the concrete stage of thinking throughout their secondary education. The TGAT Report (1987) noted that there is a seven year range of attainment at Key Stage 3 (14 years). This ability for abstract reasoning also affects other aspects of the young person's development. Adolescents are constantly challenging adult values and decisions and they begin to think about abstract concepts such as freedom and justice and formulate their own views. Many teenagers enter a period of idealism when they want to change the world and put right the mistakes of the previous generation.

From the viewpoint of the adult who is counselling an adolescent, they are much easier to communicate with as their language and thought processes are nearer those of the adult. However, it is still important to check out carefully that what is being communicated is understood and not to assume that their apparent sophistication is real.

Social and emotional development

Adolescents become absorbed with themselves at this period of development and they are always evaluating themselves in terms of other people's reactions. They are extremely self-conscious and often believe that their thoughts and feelings are unique and cannot be understood by adults. 'Who am I?' becomes an important question and various persona are tried out for size. There are various developmental tasks for the adolescent to complete and by using the list provided by Havighurst we can see how these tasks are achieved:

1. Acquire more mature social skills;
2. Achieve a masculine or feminine gender role;
3. Accept the change in one's body and one's physique and use one's body effectively;
4. Achieve emotional independence from parents and other adults;
5. Prepare for sex, marriage and parenthood;
6. Select and prepare for an occupation;
7. Develop a personal ideology and ethical standards;
8. Assume membership in the larger community.

(Havighurst R, *Developmental Tasks and Education* 1972)

This is a formidable list of tasks to be achieved and of course some adolescents are more successful than others in reaching these goals. For the abused adolescent, these tasks can present particular difficulties and these will be considered under the individual headings which have relevance for counselling.

Acquire more mature social skills

'For most boys and girls, the transition from childhood into adolescence is marked by trading a dependency on their parents to a dependency on their peers' (Steinberg and Silverberg 1986). The influence of the peer group assumes great importance at this stage and between the ages of 12 and 14 years, this influence is at its peak. Adolescents typically prefer the company of their friends to that of adults and they spend more time talking to their peers than in any other single activity (Czikszentmihalyi and Larson 1984). They also describe themselves as most happy when engaged in these interactions. Many parents of adolescents will be able to identify with this finding as one frequent source of conflict in the home is the amount of time adolescents spend on the telephone talking to their friends even when they have just parted from them. In the early stages of adolescence, friendship groups are still mainly same sex but increased contact soon develops with groups of the opposite sex as a precursor to individual dating. Among teenagers, physical attractiveness is an important factor in popularity especially with the opposite sex, and they are keenly aware of this. There is a strong urge toward group conformity in such matters as hairstyle, clothing and taste in music and it is important for acceptance not to stand out from one's peers. Adolescent friendships are relatively stable in nature although the nature of these friendships varies between the sexes. Girls tend to associate in smaller groups and develop more intimate relationships with their friends, based on the sharing of personal thoughts and feelings. This intimacy can cause problems when disagreements occur as the sense of betrayal is greater when confidences are shared with others without permission. Boys' friendships, on the other hand, are more fluid and tend to be based around shared interests.

Many researchers have noted that those who have been sexually abused frequently have poor social skills due to their low self-image. They view themselves in such negative terms as 'dirty and disgusting' and cannot imagine that they could be valued by their peer group. Their sexual abuse also isolates them from the shared experiences of their peers as they have a secret which they cannot share. When they do disclose, the reactions of the peer group are sometimes less than sympathetic or understanding. This confirms the victims in their feeling of isolation. Sometimes their efforts to form friendships have disastrous outcomes and result in further abuse as they feel powerless and unable to be assertive on their own behalf. Some girls may become promiscuous in an attempt to prove to themselves and others that they are desirable. However, by acting in such a sexual manner, society condemns them further and sees them as being responsible for their own victimisation. Boys on the other hand may act out in an anti-social or aggressive manner which further alienates them from their peer group. This behaviour is often dealt with in a punitive manner and is not seen as a possible sign that the boy has been abused.

Since acceptance by one's peers is such an important aspect of the adolescent years, having no friends or being rejected by the group has serious consequences for the development of young people's social skills and view of themselves.

Achieve a masculine or feminine gender role
We have seen in earlier chapters how gender roles become established gradually over the first six to eight years of a child's life and once these roles are established they are deeply held and often difficult to change. The male stereotype seems to develop earlier and can be stronger than the female stereotype, perhaps because children see women in a greater variety of roles during the early years (e.g. mother, teacher, school doctor etc). Masculine traits are more valued in society (Broverman et al 1970) as it is seen as good to be independent, assertive, logical and strong. Those girls who view themselves as possessing some masculine traits are likely to have higher self-esteem than those who adopt the more traditional female stereotype. Parents have a powerful influence in the establishment of these gender roles when they reward behaviours they see as sex appropriate and punish those which are inappropriate. Fathers are apparently less comfortable with girlish behaviour in their sons and are more likely to disapprove of this than they are with tomboyish behaviour in their daughters (Bee 1989). By the time adolescence is reached, gender roles are firmly established and, although some blurring occurs, many of these beliefs continue to influence us in adult life. The differing gender roles of male and female are clearly laid down in our culture and although we pay lip service to the concept of equality between the genders, the reality is often very different. The same trait is viewed very differently depending on the gender, e.g. a man may be described as assertive whereas the same behaviour in a woman is more likely to be labelled aggressive.

Abused adolescents receive powerful messages from these gender role stereotypes as to how they should regard themselves. Boys have historically been seen as less vulnerable to sexual abuse due to the limited numbers who appear in the statistics. However, it is now beginning to be acknowledged that the size of the problem of male victims has been greatly underestimated. 'It does seem that the

meaning attached to gender in our society may well underpin why boys
are less likely to be recognised as abused and to report their abuse'
(Peake 1988). The male stereotype does not envisage the boy as a
victim as males are expected to be able to take care of themselves and
retaliate to any assault. 'Society's definition of masculinity does not
expect males to express feelings of dependency, fear, vulnerability or
helplessness' (Nasjleti 1980). It is small wonder 'that male victims
report that they feel they should have been in control of the situation
and are ashamed to have been a victim' (Monaco and Gaier 1988). If
the possibility of males being victims is not part of our gender concept
then it should not surprise us that males find it so difficult to disclose
abuse and feel that their situation is so unusual that it will not be
credible.

These gender stereotypes are reflected in the differing views of what
is appropriate sexual behaviour in young males and females. The
sexual exploits of the male are often dismissed as natural and 'what
boys do'. The attitude towards the female who is sexually active at an
early age is very different and derogatory labels are often attached to
her, such as slut, whore, slag. If boys are expected to be sexually active
then this can leave the sexually abused victim unclear as to whether
what happened was really abuse or just part of becoming a man. As
parents often do not think of their male children as being in danger of
possible sexual assault, they do not warn them of such a possibility.
This lack of information can further confuse boys and make them
unsure about what has happened to them.

Although the female gender stereotype is less rigid than the male
one, the abused teenage girl may learn through her experiences that
she is only valued in terms of her sexuality and her ability to meet the
needs of the male. She may respond in a passive and victim like manner
or resort to hostile acting out behaviour which further alienates her
from adults and her peers.

Accept the change in one's body and one's physique
and use one's body effectively

The adolescent's body is changing rapidly during this period with the
development of secondary sexual characteristics and a complex
sequence of hormonal changes. They become preoccupied with their
appearance and spend hours in the bathroom and looking at
themselves in mirrors to achieve the right effect. As their body parts
grow at differing rates, adolescents often appear awkward and badly
coordinated. Those whose physical development proceeds at a slower
rate become anxious as to whether they are normal and this affects
their self confidence and image of themselves. Fashions as to the ideal
body shape are transmitted by our culture and girls in particular are
anxious to acquire the shape that is currently in vogue. This can lead to

anxieties about being too fat and experimenting with various diets. For overweight children between the ages of 11 and 17, the relationship between self-esteem and body esteem is closely linked (Mendelson and White 1985). Overweight boys suffer a low self-esteem between the ages of 11 and 13 while overweight girls' self-esteem suffers more in late adolescence. In extreme cases this can lead to adolescents developing anorexia nervosa with the risk of possible death unless treatment is successful.

Other factors in society militate against adolescents using their bodies effectively and not abusing them. In an attempt to acquire the outward signs of maturity, teenagers become involved in smoking, drinking and substance abuse. As adolescence is a time of risk taking, health education promotions are often ignored and regarded as irrelevant.

Many teenage girls who have been sexually abused see themselves as 'damaged goods' (Sgroi) and fear they have become physically damaged, especially if the experience was a painful one. They frequently seek reassurance that their bodies are normal and that they will be able to produce normal children in the future. These fears can often be reduced following disclosure if they are acknowledged and dealt with by a sensitive medical examination. This image of being damaged can be reinforced by society's response following disclosure. If the case is covered by the media, the victims often become a source of curiosity to the peer group who may put pressure on them for details of what happened. Others may view the victims as available and make sexual propositions to them leading to the possibility of further abuse. Some abused teenagers feel that their body has betrayed them, especially if they have been sexually aroused by the experience. As male victims are often faced with visible evidence of a physical response to the abuse, i.e. an erection, they can become confused as to whether they wanted the initial contact or not and were willing partners rather than victims. This feeling of responsibility for their own abuse can lead to self-abusive behaviours towards their own bodies, i.e. cutting themselves with razors or knives, alcohol and drug abuse and suicide attempts. The following case illustrates many of these points:

> Brenda was an academically able girl who first came to notice through her frequent bouts of drunken behaviour and involvement in the local drug scene. In spite of efforts to help her with these problems, her behaviour deteriorated and she became desperately anorexic. She would wear baggy clothes to hide her female shape and to disguise the fact that she was losing weight rapidly. She went to great lengths to pretend that she was eating normally and saw herself as ugly and 'too fat'. She was unable to look at her body while bathing and avoided seeing herself in a mirror. Brenda made several serious attempts at suicide, both before and after she disclosed her abusive experience and clearly hated her body which she saw as having betrayed her.

Achieve emotional independence from parents and other adults

The teenage years give rise to an increased conflict with parents and other adults in authority as young people attempt to become individuals in their own right. Authority is constantly being challenged and adolescents become more critical of their parents and are quick to note that adults often behave in ways which are contrary to the standards set for them. *The Secret Diary of Adrian Mole* (Townsend 1982) contains many amusing illustrations of the teenager's often perceptive view of adults and their behaviour:

> My mother is looking for a job! Now I could end up a delinquent roaming the streets and all that... I will be a latchkey kid, whatever that is... I will be forced to eat crisps and sweets until my skin is ruined and my teeth fall out. I think my mother is being very selfish. She won't be any good in a job anyway. She isn't very bright and she drinks too much at Christmas.

This quotation illustrates beautifully, the adolescent's preoccupation with themselves.

Pressures from the peer group can exacerbate these conflicts with parents and most arguments arise over dress, music, hairstyle and limitations placed on their freedom. Often teenagers feel overcriticised by their parents and complain that their opinions are not considered or even listened to during discussions. However, in spite of these areas of conflict, most adolescents want their parents to be interested in them, and it is essential that parents maintain their authority while allowing the adolescent a greater say. The gap between parents and teenagers is not as wide as it may appear at first glance and adolescents are likely to adopt their parents' views on broader social and political issues.

As most adolescents are moving towards greater independence, abused teenagers can often find themselves in a dependency trap. When abuse occurs within the family, many abused girls are prevented from engaging in normal social contacts and dating, due to the jealousy of the perpetrator. They are warned that boys are only after 'one thing' and are discouraged from the usual boy/girl relationships. The teenager increasingly resents these restrictions on her social life and frequently discloses abuse as a result of a row over these restrictions. In addition, some sexually abused girls assume an adult role within the family, taking over the responsibilities of the mother in running the house and looking after younger children as well as being a sexual partner for father. This further restricts social contact with her peers and she becomes more and more isolated and unable to break away and achieve independence. Boys are typically allowed more freedom to take part in social activities and may fear that if they do tell of an abusive incident their freedom will be restricted in the future.

Prepare for sex, marriage and parenthood

Sexual interest and behaviour increases sharply with the physical and hormonal changes occurring in the teenagers's body. The development of secondary sex characteristics makes us aware that sexual maturity is approaching and teenagers are often embarrassed by their lack of control over their bodies at this time. Masturbation in private continues with increased frequency and pornographic magazines are much prized by boys and circulate freely. As interest in the opposite sex develops, much experimentation occurs and this is a topic for discussion and often bragging in same sex friendship groups. Advertising and the media increasingly encourage younger adolescents to behave in ways more appropriate to an older age group, and the preadolescent child is increasingly being targeted for fashionable clothes with sexual overtones. Adolescents are interested in viewing other's bodies, especially those of the opposite sex, and voyeuristic behaviour such as looking in changing room windows is common. Malmquist states that 'the most common type of sexual behaviour in adolescents after masturbation, is probably heterosexual contact with another adolescent (1985 p.37).

It is of course true that some teenagers have same-sex sexual interaction with their peers, but this does not necessarily reflect an adolescent's sexual identity or preference. An increased interest in sex and sexual experimentation within one's peer group is therefore the norm for most adolescents. Although more teenagers are sexually active earlier and with a greater number of partners, promiscuous behaviour is disapproved of by most adolescents. However, teenagers do reflect society's views on this matter, being more critical of girls who have many partners than they are of boys. This is illustrated by the greater number of abusive terms used for girls such as 'slut', 'slag', 'whore', whereas boys are described by terms such as 'stud' which have more positive connotations.

Making decisions about their sexuality and sexual behaviour is extremely important for the adolescent, but for those who have been victims of sexual abuse:

> the decisions have already been made regardless of the adolescent's desires. Often sexual abuse has occurred at a previous time when no choice or right to protection existed.
>
> (Hindman 1989)

Whereas most adolescents are looking forward towards sexual fulfilment, the abused victim is constantly looking back with feelings of guilt and shame.

Sexual experimentation can trigger off frightening or painful memories and this may lead the adolescent to avoid all sexual contact.

Some abused girls find that they are unable to tolerate any form of physical contact with a boy as they immediately experience flashbacks of their abuse. Others may see sexuality as a means to meeting others needs, such as acceptance by the peer group and they behave in a promiscuous manner feeling their body has no value.

> Margaret was a seriously abused teenager who had suffered sexual, physical and emotional abuse from her father from the age of 7 years. She had few friends as she was not allowed any social contact with her peers apart from school. At the age of 15 years, having been received into care, she was allowed, for the first time, to take part in social activities. However, when a boy invited her to a disco and bought her crisps and a coke, she felt under an obligation to offer him sexual favours in return. She had learned all too well the deadly lesson that she had to pay for any pleasure!

Many abused girls have anxieties about marriage and having children as they fear they will be unable to protect their children just as their mothers were unable to protect them. Having experienced abuse they feel unable to be assertive on their own behalf and are therefore vulnerable to becoming involved in further abusive situations.

For male victims, being sexually abused by another male can cause difficulties over their concept of themselves as a sexual being. In attempting to understand why he was selected by the perpetrator, the boy victim may assume that he was chosen because of his personal characteristics. He fears that others see him as feminine and therefore he must be so. The fact that he was unable to resist the abuse may be internalised as an indication that he is not really a man. If the experience has been pleasurable, then this reinforces his anxiety over his sexual identity and confirms his fear that he must be homosexual.

Some boys attempt to deal with these feelings by reasserting their masculinity through aggressive behaviour, since aggression is regarded as a masculine trait. In addition, if he presents a tough image to the world he may feel that this will protect him from abuse in the future. This desire for reasserting his own masculinity and being in control can lead some male victims to sexually abuse other children. 'In its most common form, the apparent need of the boy victim to reenact his own victimisation appears to be but a variation upon inappropriate attempts to reassert his own masculinity' (Rogers and Terry). Male victims typically find it difficult to discuss their molestation or their feelings, and generally just want to forget it ever happened:

> The inability of many of these victim/offender boys to empathise with their victims may reflect a denial process in which the child essentially denies his own experience and his own feelings.
>
> (Rogers and Terry)

Develop a personal ideology and ethical standards

We have seen how throughout childhood decisions about goodness and badness, right and wrong, have been formulated according to the developmental stage a child has reached. By the time adolescence is reached, moral judgements are made on a basis closer to that of the adult. Kohlberg referred to this level as 'conventional morality'. Judgements are based on the premise of maintaining good relations with others and winning their approval and issues of right and wrong tend to be evaluated in terms of conformity to society's rules and regulations. Although adolescents are aware of the rules of society, it does not always follow that they will abide by them. Much of the risk taking behaviour so typical of adolescents brings them into conflict with these rules and inevitably some are broken. On occasion, the rights of the individual may conflict with the rules laid down by society. The individual has to solve these dilemmas by operating at a higher level of moral development, where evaluation is based on one's own belief system instead of blind conformity to the expectations of society or the group. This is clearly a mature level of operation which many adolescents and adults do not attain. In the early stages of establishing a value system, many adolescents are attracted to ideologies and religious cults which are rather rigid and authoritarian. These may serve the purpose of helping the adolescent to know where they stand and what is important in life. However, as they become more confident of their own points of view, some are able to dispense with these systems and adopt a more personal standpoint.

> Moral development is clearly affected by sexually abusive experiences. Clinical experience indicates this is not always in a negative way. Many children who have been sexually abused show a very highly developed sense of what is right, wrong, just or fair. This rather seems to be because they have had to make their own evaluation based on their experiences of sexual abuse... They know that you cannot tell what someone is like merely by looking at them.
>
> (Smith).

Often the perpetrator is someone who is well regarded by the community and may claim to have sound moral values. If the case is not proceeded with, or the perpetrator is cleared of all charges in court, what message does the adolescent learn about morality? Can we be surprised if they are confused as to what is right and what is wrong?

Codes of values can give deadly messages to victims of sexual abuse as they are all too ready to view themselves as sinners and responsible for their own abuse. Girls who are raised in cultures which place high value on the virginity and sexual purity of females before marriage see themselves, and may be seen by others, as soiled and unworthy as a result of their abusive experiences.

The adolescent and HIV/AIDS

Due to increased media coverage and health promotion education about HIV/AIDS in schools, many adolescents are aware of the existence of AIDS in the community at large. In addition many of the risk activities teenagers indulge in, such as drug substance abuse, promiscuity, running away from home or living on the streets, place them in a position of heightened risk of possible infection. This is especially true for those who have been abused. However, there is still evidence of a great deal of misinformation about the subject amongst teenagers, as in the general adult population, and this needs to be addressed. 'The major aspect of HIV/AIDS in all ages is the effect on relationships' (Miller et al 1989). As teenagers are most concerned about the image others have of them, having to deal with the possibility of being HIV positive can have a major impact on them developmentally. How to deal with this situation will be discussed in detail in section 3 of this book. For the sexually abused adolescent, coping with the possibility of a life threatening illness in addition to the sequelae of abuse may well increase their symptoms of poor self-esteem, guilt, blame, stigma, and isolation. As Honigsbaum states:

> some staff working with very emotionally damaged teenage girls have counselled against testing as fear, self-loathing and depression can be reinforced — and it can even precipitate a young person into suicide and self-destructive behaviour.

These risks have to be evaluated by the AIDS counsellor as have the effects on the family should the child prove HIV positive. Those adolescents who present for counselling will need help and guidance in relation to their own sexuality and how being HIV+ will affect their sexual and social relationships. With younger children the counsellor will have to tackle issues such as when, how and if to tell the child, what to tell siblings and how to maintain hope in the face of a life threatening illness.

Summary

- Important physical, emotional and social changes occur during the period of adolescence and a range of developmental tasks have to be undertaken to enable the adolescent to achieve adult status.

- The peer group is highly influential and there is a strong urge to group conformity. Many sexually abused adolescents have poor social skills and rejection by the peer group can lead to dysfunctional behaviour.

- Society has different expectations for the gender roles of male and females. The male stereotype does not envisage boys as victims, making it more difficult for them to admit to abuse. Female victims can be blamed for their own victimisation and may see themselves as valued only for their sexual qualities.

- Acquiring a positive body image is important for the adolescent's self-esteem. Those who have been sexually abused may view their bodies in negative terms leading to self mutilation and abuse.

- For the adolescent to achieve maturity, they must gain emotional independence from adults by challenging adult authority. Girls who have been sexually abused may be prevented from achieving independence by emotional ties to the perpetrator.

- The development of heterosexual relationships and increased sexual experimentation can pose problems for sexually abused teenagers. Girls may see themselves as damaged goods and avoid sexual contact or become promiscuous. Males may fear they are homosexual and resort to attempts to reassert their masculinity through aggressive behaviour or reenacting their own victimisation.

- Although some sexually abused adolescents have a highly developed sense of moral values, the double standards operating in society can cause confusion about what is right and wrong.

- The possibility of acquiring a life threatening infection as a result of sexual abuse is likely to compound the existing damage and is increasingly becoming an issue for those who have been abused.

References

Bee H, 1989 *The developing child* 5th edn. Harper Collins, New York.

Broverman I K, Broverman D, Clarkson F E, Rosenkrantz P S, Vogel S R, 1970 Sex-role stereotypes and clinical judgements of mental health. *Journal of consulting and clinical psychology* **34**: 1–7.

Czikszentmihalyi M, Larson R, 1984 *Being adolescent: conflict and growth in the teenage years.* Basic Books, New York, US.

Havighurst R, 1972 *Developmental tasks and education.* David McKay, New York, US.

Hindman J, 1989 *Just before dawn.* Alexandria Associates, Oregon.

Honigsbaum N, 1991 *HIV, AIDS and children, a cause for concern.* National Childrens Bureau.

Malmquist C P, 1985 Sexual offences among adolescents. *Medical aspects of human sexuality* **19** (9): 134–39.

Mendelson B, White D, 1985 Development of self-body esteem in overweight youngsters. *Developmental psychology* **21**: 90–96.

Miller R, Goldman R, Bor R, Kernoff P, 1989 AIDS and children: some of the issues in haemophilia care and how to address them. *AIDS care* **1** (1).

Monaco N M, Gaier E L, 1988 Differential patterns of disclosure of child abuse among boys and girls: implications for practitioners. *Early child development and care* **30**: 97–103.

Nasjleti M, 1980 Suffering in Silence: the male incest victim. *Child Welfare* **LIX** (5).

Peake A, 1988 *Issues of under-reporting: the sexual abuse of boys.* Paper presented at British Psychological Society Annual Conference.

Rogers C M, Terry T, 1982 Clinical intervention with boy victims of sexual abuse. In Stuart I R, Greer J G (eds) *Victims of sexual aggression: treatment of children, women and men.* Van Nostrand Reinhold, New York, US.

Sgroi S M, 1982 *Handbook of clinical intervention in child sexual abuse.* Lexington Books, Massachussetts, US.

Smith G, 1992 In V. P. Varma (ed) *The secret life of vulnerable children.* Routledge, London

Steinberg L, Silverberg S, 1986 The vicissitudes of autonomy in early adolescence. *Child development* **57**: 841–51.

TGAT (Task Group on Assessment and Testing), 1987 (report) Department of Education and Science and The Welsh Office.

Townsend S, 1982 *The secret diary of Adrian Mole aged 13.* Methuen.

4 Sex rings

Introduction

The choice of the title 'sex rings' for this chapter has been a deliberate one and this term is used in preference to 'network or organised abuse' and 'multiple abuse situations', which have gained popularity in recent times. These terms were rejected on the grounds that they could give rise to misunderstanding and did not adequately describe the situations discussed in this chapter. Not all sex rings are organised or operate as a network although some undoubtedly do, and the term does not cover what Burgess (Burgess et al 1981), described as solo rings. The title multiple abuse situation also poses problems as some children are multiply abused by several perpetrators over a period of time, but not necessarily in the company of other children.

Most research into child sexual abuse has focused on the area of interfamilial abuse. Abuse by perpetrators who are outside the family has received less attention. The effects for the victim of 'stranger abuse' are generally regarded as being less traumatic and severe, due to the fact that the child is able to receive support from the family after disclosure. However, in recent years many examples of child sex rings have been reported in the media with one containing as many as 400 preschool children. Children who are abused in this manner have clearly an increased risk of becoming infected not only with sexually transmitted diseases, but also with the HIV virus. It would appear that we have to take on board that prolonged sexual abuse of large numbers of children may be common (Wild and Wynne 1986). Recently, three such rings came to light in Cornwall and the effects of these on the victims and their families will be discussed in this chapter with some suggestions about therapeutic interventions.

What is a sex ring?

Burgess et al (1981) describe a sex ring as 'a situation in which at least one offender is simultaneously involved with several victims, all of whom are aware of the other's participation'. These rings can be categorised into three types, solo, transitional and syndicated.

Solo ring
This consists of one adult who is sexually involved with small groups of children. The ring usually operates on its own and does not have links with other rings.

Transitional ring
In this type of ring, several adults are involved with groups of children and there may be periodic contact with other paedophiles and their groups.

Syndicated ring
These rings involve several adults in a well structured organisation designed to recruit children for the provision of pornography and other sexual services. The syndicated rings have a wide network of customers and pornographic material is freely distributed for gain.

Pornography is widely used in all types of sex rings but does not always involve the children in the ring. When a large ring in London was uncovered, pornography was discovered which led to connections with a ring of perpetrators in Cornwall.

How do the perpetrators operate?

Offenders who are involved in sex rings are usually male and may be of any age. In the 11 rings identified in Leeds, the perpetrators ranged in age from 30 to 82. Older adolescents usually leave the ring when they are no longer of interest to the paedophiles running the group, but some remain and take on the role of a perpetrator.

In sex rings, the child's cooperation in sexual acts is gained by the use of bribery, manipulation and enticement. These men may frequent such places as amusement arcades or fairgrounds, where children are known to gather, or gain access to children through positions of authority in legitimate children's groups such as youth clubs, Scout groups and children's homes. Perpetrators often go to great lengths to make themselves known to the children's parents and gain their trust by appearing helpful and responsible adults, and legitimising their interest in their children. One such offender in a Cornish ring always asked permission from the parents when he took the children on treats and made sure the children were returned at the time stated. He offered to look after the children to enable parents to go out for the evening, and gained their sympathy by telling them about the hard life he had endured.

Another perpetrator became a family friend and gave them a gift of money when they were in financial difficulties. When the abuser has a good reputation in the community or occupies a position of authority, this makes it more difficult for any allegation of sexual abuse to be believed.

Once children have become involved with the perpetrator, they are often used to recruit others. This was noted in several of the larger rings in Leeds where children who acted as ringleaders and deputies were identified. In the girls ring in Cornwall, one girl who had known the abuser since she was four years old held a powerful position within the group and controlled who had treats and who was invited to join the group.

After children are introduced into the ring their continued cooperation and loyalty is ensured by various means. Bribery is a common feature as the children who cooperate are rewarded with money, special treats and privileges. Often the children will vie with each other for the adult's attention and approval. Secrecy is essential if the activities of the ring are to continue and this is achieved by threats, peer pressure and blackmail. Many victims are afraid of telling because of threats which have been made or implied. As one boy stated 'X could get you to do things and you wouldn't realise you were doing it. If you didn't he could turn nasty'. Often children are introduced to other illegal activities such as alcohol, cigarettes and drugs and these can be used to blackmail them into secrecy. One boy was more concerned about his parents finding out that he was smoking than taking part in the sexual activities. The pressure of the peer group is very important in maintaining loyalty to the offender and the group, and involving children in sexual activities with each other reinforces their view of themselves as willing participants. The pressures to ensure secrecy are so effective that even when a perpetrator has been apprehended, many victims are unwilling to tell what happened.

How are rings discovered?

Both boys and girls can be involved in sex rings and rings are either single sex or mixed. In general their ages range between six and 14 years, although some rings contain preschool children and older adolescents.

In the Leeds rings the vast majority of the victims were girls (171 out of 175) whereas the London rings were made up of boys. In Cornwall, there were two boys rings and one girls ring. The existence of these rings is often discovered accidentally as when members of the public report large numbers of children going to the homes of unattached men or victims run away from home. The Leeds rings were discovered when one girl attempted to castrate a young boy when she was baby-sitting, claiming that she was 'fed up with willies' (Campbell 1988: p.104). In Cornwall the girls' ring came to light when three of the youngsters told an ancillary at school after watching a video about good and bad secrets. One of the boys' rings was disclosed when two social workers called at the wrong address on another investigation.

The initial investigation of a ring is a time consuming business and many continue for many months. Both the police and social service departments can be placed under great stress to provide adequate resources to cope with the work load. It is essential that the investigation of sex rings is seen as a child protection issue and not a straightforward criminal investigation. Initial interviews need to be conducted by police and social workers who are aware of the dynamics of sexual abuse, as a high level of resistance is often encountered when questioning alleged victims. The pressures to maintain the secret and fear of possible retribution from the perpetrator or other members of the group all militate against the investigation of the ring.

Effects on victims

Before disclosure, children involved in the rings often appear to have symptoms similar to other forms of sexual abuse, i.e. physical complaints, anxiety symptoms, behavioural difficulties. Following disclosure, many parents report increased difficulty in coping with their children's challenging and acting out behaviour. In one of the boys' groups in Cornwall there was an increase in disruptive behaviour both at home and at school, with some children becoming withdrawn, while others indulged in antisocial behaviour and emotional outbursts. For those children whose behaviour had been problematical before involvement in the ring, disclosure appeared to heighten these difficulties.

Burgess et al (1984) conducted a follow-up study two years after rings were exposed in order to assess whether long term effects were evident. She categorised four patterns of response from her findings which she labelled *integration of the event; avoidance of the event; repetition of symptoms; and identification with the exploiter.* Three quarters of the sample were deemed to have continuing difficulties.

Integration of the event
Those who were able to integrate the experience could discuss what happened, had reduced anxiety and were able to place the responsibility for the abusive activities with the perpetrator. They were also able to resume a normal lifestyle and look towards the future.

Avoidance of the event
These children refused to discuss what had happened, feeling that it

was better forgotten and put behind them. They had suppressed their anxieties but retained fear of the perpetrator.

Repetition of symptoms
In this category, victims resembled those suffering from acute post traumatic stress disorder, experiencing feelings of guilt and self blame for having participated in the ring.

Identification with the exploiter
Those children who identified with the exploiter dealt with their anxieties by minimising what had happened and exploiting others. Victims in this group had difficulty with authority figures, remained attached emotionally to the offender and indulged in antisocial behaviour.

Both in the American studies and in Leeds acting out behaviour learned in the sex rings was common. Those who participated for a long time in the ring, or who had been involved in pornography for gain appeared to be at the greatest risk of serious long term effects.

It is too soon to consider the long term effects for children involved in the Cornish rings, but many of the behaviours listed have been noted. Many of the boys were reluctant to admit their involvement ('nothing happened to me', 'I didn't see anything'), or minimised their participation ('I only watched a video', 'he never touched me'). As this minimisation was often reinforced by those parents who just wanted to forget about it, engaging these boys in a therapeutic programme proved impossible. One of the boys was angry about the conviction of the offender and threatened to beat up the boy who had told.

How can the victims be helped?

If the findings of Burgess are correct, and the results from the Leeds ring would appear to lend support to these, therapeutic intervention to break down the secrecy is essential. Christopherson suggests that all the members of the group, with their parents, should be assembled to review what happened. This technique has certainly been effective in debriefing those involved in disaster work and it would appear to have some merit. Nevertheless, constraints placed on dealing with information which may still be sub judice may make this suggestion difficult to carry out. However, the fact that a matter has become *sub judice* does not create an absolute ban on saying anything. The real danger lies in the child being given information or having the facts of the case discussed with him/her in a way which might influence the evidence the child ultimately gives to court (White 1987). Experience that intervention is most effective at the point of crisis and delay enables victims and their families to deal with the situation in a dysfunctional manner. The longer the period of delay, the more difficult it is to engage them in a therapeutic programme. A possible solution to this dilemma will be discussed in the second part of this chapter. Some victims in sex rings may show marked behavioural or psychological problems which will require intensive individual help and it would be helpful to have some form of screening device which could enable these victims to be identified.

Due to the numbers involved, group work would appear to be the most effective means of dealing with the majority of victims. However, these groups can prove difficult to handle as there is a strong element of secrecy within the group and a group cohesiveness due to its previous existence within the ring. Boys in particular find it difficult to talk about their abuse and the feelings connected with the experience but those abused in a sex ring may have additional constraints about sharing their experiences in the presence of other members of the ring.

Once permission to break the secrecy and to talk openly about what happened to them has been established the following issues need to be addressed in groups for victims abused in sex rings:

● To learn and develop the skills essential for self-protection in the future;

● How perpetrators operate, in order to reduce their feelings of self-blame and responsibility for the abuse;

● Feelings towards the perpetrators, both positive and negative;

● Normal sexual development and confusion about their own sexuality (e.g. homosexuality);

● Rebuilding self-esteem and developing control over one's life in order to counter helplessness and victimisation;

● Reestablishing normal group relationships with peers;

● Why children cannot tell — nature of the violence/pressures involved;

● Dealing with sexualised behaviour patterns;

● Fears of being an abuser;

● AIDS/HIV   This topic is best dealt with initially by means of individual counselling sessions before being addressed in a group setting.

Some items are common to groups of both sexes, while others are particular to the needs of boys.

Effects of the discovery of sex rings on victims' families

When children are sexually abused by a person outside the family, the anguish of their parents may be more immediately acute than that of the children. To the parents, the news is surprising and shocking, whereas the children have been living with the information for some time and have accommodated it. As the family's reaction to the discovery of assault strongly affects the impact of the abuse on the child (Pelletier and Handy 1986), help for parents is essential.

Parents show a wide variation in their reactions when confronted about their child's involvement in a sex ring. They have to deal with their own powerful feelings while trying to support their children, and if they do not receive help, the effects of the abuse on the children can be compounded. The responses noted below were found by Regehr (1990) and Burgess (1981) and were confirmed by the findings from the Cornish rings.

Surprise and disbelief
Frequently, parents are totally surprised when the news is first broken to them and they are often unable to believe what has happened. This is particularly true when the offender is well respected and has a position of authority in the community. Their disbelief may cause them to question the truthfulness of their children's allegations as they are unable to believe that such a caring and helpful person would do such things to children. If the parents knew the offender well and had encouraged his access to their child, this makes matters worse. Other parents are less surprised and admit to the fact that they were suspicious of him ('you never saw him with other adults, he was always hanging around with a crowd of kids', 'I always thought there was something funny about him').

Anger
Anger and the urge for retaliation is very common especially among fathers and they often voice what they would like to do to the offender if they could get their hands on him, ('just give me 10 minutes with him and I'd sort him out', 'hanging is too good for him'). This anger often spills over on to the victim and 'parents are often angry at some level towards their child for not preventing the abuse, for not telling the parents about it, for disrupting the parents' lives' (Regehr 1990). When several children in the family are involved, the blame may be directed at the eldest for not protecting the younger ones. If the children are teenagers, parents may wonder whether they in fact consented to what happened and fathers in particular may wonder whether their sons have homosexual tendencies. Although anger is a frequent response from parents, some are more ambivalent in their reactions and

maintain they feel sorry for the offender and don't wish to bring charges against him. This attitude can give a powerful message to the victim whose feelings of self-blame are reinforced.

Anger can also be directed towards the system, especially if parents feel that matters have not been handled properly by the authorities. If the offender escapes punishment either by disappearing, or by being found not guilty in court, this can leave parents feeling powerless and frustrated. When the media report details of the sex rings, parents are often angry at the insensitive manner in which this is done, especially if the reports enable the victims or their families to be identified by the rest of the community.

Guilt
Feelings of guilt are extremely common as parents feel that at some level they must be to blame. These responses are strengthened if they willingly gave consent for their children to be with the offender and knew and trusted him. Society tends to believe that if children are sexually abused the parents are in part responsible, and this is reinforced by the professional literature where we find comments such as 'marital conflicts, parental absences and family disruption are strongly related to extra familial child sexual assault' (Sgroi 1982). Some parents readily assume responsibility for what happened, feeling that they have failed as parents because they did not adequately supervise their children or check out the offender. These feelings can be compounded if the system does not handle distressed parents in a sympathetic manner and conveys, even indirectly, the attitude that what happened is to some extent the fault of the parents. As a result of these feelings of responsibility, parents feel shame and embarrassment at what happened to their child and are unable to share the information with their normal support group of friends and family.

Minimising
Hearing what has happened to their child is often so painful that parents attempt to cope with the pain by minimising their child's part in the activities of the ring. As children often fear the reaction of their parents to what has happened, they may either deny being involved or give a limited account of what happened to them. Some parents do not wish to hear the details and the child responds accordingly. If a child denies involvement when interviewed, parents often do not wish the child to be subjected to further questioning even if there are considerable grounds for believing that the child was actively involved.

Many of these feelings get in the way of parents being able to support their child and enabling them to meet other parents in the same situation can be a therapeutic experience. Parents need help for themselves as well as advice on how to help their children. This can be done on an individual basis at the time of the investigation, or by means of a group where they are able to share their experiences and regain control over what is happening to them. The following issues need to be addressed in parent groups:

- Parents need an opportunity to vent their conflicting feelings without the child being present. By sharing with others how they feel about what has happened, they come to understand that they are not alone and the feelings they are experiencing are usual and to be expected.

- The issue of guilt needs to be tackled to enable them to absolve themselves of unjustifiable self-blame. As with the victims group, they need to place the responsibility with the offender, while making them more aware of the potential dangers to their child.

- Parents need to learn how to handle the behavioural difficulties which may face them once the abuse has come to light. This was a high priority with the parents in one group who expressed fears about damaging the child further. They need help in establishing reasonable limits and dealing with inappropriate behaviour in a calm and sensible manner. By learning how children are likely to respond to abuse, i.e. what is normal and what should give rise for concern, parents can begin to feel in control again and start to put their lives back together. They need to know where they can get help for themselves and their children if problems persist.

- The need for information is often high on the agenda in a parents' group. They need information about what has happened, how things will be handled, how to cope with the media, dealing with anxieties about court proceedings etc. Once an investigation takes off parents often feel they are left in the dark and, as delays are usual, this increases their anxiety and feelings of helplessness and isolation.

- Feelings towards the victims. It is vital that parents' feelings towards the victim are addressed if the child is not to be further traumatised. When parents feel that it is best forgotten, the child does not have permission to talk about the abuse. This reinforces their feeling that something so dreadful has happened to them that it cannot be spoken about. Anger directed towards the child for not preventing the abuse or not telling the parents ('why couldn't he tell me?', 'why did he keep going back when he knew what was happening?') can prevent parents helping their child. By learning how perpetrators operate and the pressures and threats which militate against children telling, parents can begin to deal with their feelings and not project them on to the child. Parents often have difficulty understanding why their child retains positive feelings towards the perpetrator after the abuse and they need to understand why this occurs. Issues of consent are also troublesome to parents. They need help in understanding the power dynamics present in sexual activity with an adult.

● Many parents find communicating with their child about the abuse extremely difficult and often need outside help to enable this to take place. If parents have not dealt with many of the issues detailed above then the child picks up the feelings of the parents and is unable to be open with them.

● Fears for the future. Many parents experienced fear about whether their children would be damaged in the long term as a result of what had happened to them. Will they become an abuser? Will they be at greater risk of further abuse? Will he become homo-sexual? are all typical questions in the minds of parents. These fears need to be addressed calmly by giving parents information and by suggesting ways in which they can help their child.

● AIDS/HIV Infection publicity campaigns have increased the public awareness of AIDS. Parents are increasingly anxious about the question of HIV infection, especially if their child has been involved in sex ring activities. In one group it was clear that the information parents had was incomplete and often faulty. Some parents were convinced that their children had been tested for the virus when they had undergone a medical examination, whereas others initially wanted to have their child tested, or force the perpetrator to undergo testing. To deal with these issues, an AIDS counsellor came along to the parents group and gave a presentation on the subject and dealt with the parents' questions. This proved to be a very effective way of giving the parents the information they required to make decisions about their children and to allay many of their anxieties. An open invitation was given to the parents to contact the counsellor on an individual basis at any point in the future if they had continuing concerns.

An evaluation of the group indicated that those parents involved had found the experience beneficial and they expressed sadness at its termination. They identified the following benefits:

● They no longer felt so isolated and sharing feelings had enabled them to realise that 'I'm not the only one with all these feelings'. Having established trust in each other they felt they could contact members of the group in the future for support.

● The parents acknowledged that their feelings of anger and guilt had been reduced as a result of their experiences in the group. They were reassured about their ability to be competent parents and knew where to get help if this was required.

- The parents felt they had a greater understanding of what their children had experienced and why they were unable to confide in them.

- As parents, they were more aware of the dangers their children were exposed to and the need for adequate supervision. This was particularly relevant for the parents of boys who had previously not contemplated the possibility of sexual assault as a potential danger.

When the police have apprehended perpetrators and gathered sufficient evidence to present before the courts then parents groups can be convened to deal with the issues previously discussed. However, as stated earlier in this chapter, parents often request and need help at an early stage of the proceedings when matters may still be sub judice. At this point it can be helpful to offer general guidance to parents, bearing in mind that the facts of the case cannot be discussed until the court appearance has been completed. The following issues could be addressed at such a meeting of parents:

- Parents can be helped to understand that reactions of outrage, disbelief and shock are both natural and normal. For the benefit of their child they should try to remain calm and not express their anger or pain. It can be made clear to parents that showing these feelings to the child may increase the child's guilt, both about being abused and about revealing the fact. The more matter-of-fact a parent can be, the more likely the child is to confide and share their feelings.

- The need for parents to let their children know that they are glad they have been able to talk about what has worried them and that they are believed and understood. Parents should also try to give the message that they would always be ready to listen if the child felt that there were parts of the story that had been forgotten or mixed up and which the child wished to change.

- The importance of trying not to ask questions such as 'why did you let him?', 'Why didn't you tell me before?'. These give the impression that the child is to blame. It is important that children understand that the onus of preventing sexual behaviour between adults and children always rests with the adult and that it is wrong of the adult to allow such behaviour.

- The fact that many children will need extra reassurance and comfort at the time of the disclosure. It is important to help the child feel safe and to be available to give the child extra time and attention.

- Many parents react quite naturally by wanting to overprotect their children. Unfortunately this might reinforce children's feelings of helplessness and so it is important to allow them to regain age-appropriate levels of responsibility and behaviour as soon as they seem ready.

- Many parents feel it is better to discourage children from talking about what happened so that they can forget as soon as possible. Parents should be made aware that children will recover from the experience quicker and more permanently if they are given permission to talk when they need to. This does not mean constantly questioning them, but rather listening to the child and responding at their pace.

- Although parents need to share with each other what has happened, they should be given the opportunity to think about the likely impact on their child if these discussions are conducted in the child's presence.

- Parents need to be helped to understand that children should express and retain any positive feelings they may have held about the abuser.

- Finally, parents need to be reminded not to ignore brothers and sisters if only one child in the family was abused. All the family need to know what happened and this can be a time to teach all the children about personal and sexual safety.

By dealing with these topics, parents can be helped to provide support to their children without discussion of the details of the offences, and it should provide a helpful model to reinforce positive parenting.

Summary

- In this chapter, the various types of sex rings are described with details of the kinds of strategies perpetrators adopt to attract children and maintain their cooperation and secrecy.

- These rings are often discovered accidentally and their investigation places great strain on the resources of the police and social service departments.

- It is clear from the research that the victims can suffer long term effects as a result of this type of sexual assault.

- It is essential that help is offered, both to the victims and their parents, if the resultant trauma is to be minimised.

- Group work would appear to be the most effective and viable way of coping with the numbers involved and suggestions are made as to the type of issues which need to be addressed.

- In both the victims' and parents' groups, the question of AIDS/HIV infection has to be dealt with in order to enable informed decisions to be made over the question of testing.

- Finally, a model is proffered for the provision of general guidance to parents at an early stage in the investigation to enable them to support their children and reinforce good parenting.

References

Burgess A W, Groth A N, McCausland M P, 1981 Child Sex Initiation Rings. *American Journal of Orthopsychiatry* **51** (1) January 1981.

Burgess A W, Hartman C R, McCausland M P, Powers P, 1984 *American Journal of Psychiatry* **141**: (5) May 1984.

Campbell B, 1988 *Unofficial secrets*. Virgo.

Christopherson J, 1989 Sex Rings. In *Working with Sexually Abused Boys* Hollows A, Armstrong H, (ed) National Children's Bureau.

Pelletier G, Handy L, 1986 Family dysfunction and the psychological impact of child sexual abuse. *Canadian Journal of Psychiatry* **31**: 407–12.

Regehr C, 1990 Parental responses to extrafamilial child sexual abuse. *Child abuse and neglect* **14**: 113–20.

Sgroi S M, 1982 *Handbook of clinical intervention in child sexual abuse.* Lexington Books. D. C. Heath & Co Massachusetts

Wild N J, Wynne J M, 1986 Child sex rings. *British Medical Journal* **293**: 183–85.

White R, 1987 *Legal opinion in child abuse in schools.* Cornwall County Council.

Section 2 CHILD SEXUAL ABUSE

Introduction

It is advisable to examine some of the many definitions of sexual abuse in order to understand the professional as opposed to lay interpretation of the phenomenon. Such an examination helps in understanding the wide range of estimates of the scope of the problem. However, it then becomes clear that the extent of the variation is a result not only of differing definitions but also of confusing incidence with prevalence. Incidence is the number of new cases in a population in one year. Prevalence is the proportion of a population who have suffered sexual abuse at any time during childhood. It must be acknowledged that another factor is the extreme difficulty victims experience in speaking of their abuse both at the time and later.

There is a wide difference between the prevalence of sexual abuse when using the figures provided by adult survivors and the incidence as illustrated by, for example, successful prosecution for sexual offences against children, or the numbers of children's names on child protection registers. The problem is further compounded by the differences between what victims and perpetrators are able to tell us at the time, as against the reality which may be made clear only many months or years later.

Counselling of victims of sexual abuse takes place within this background and it is essential that counsellors have an understanding of the secrecy which surrounds sexual abuse and the barriers this may impose.

5 Recognition of sexual abuse

Definitions
A relatively early definition of sexual abuse which has been influential in forming official opinion is that of Schechtu and Roberge (1976):

> The sexual exploitation of children refers to the involvement of dependent, developmentally immature children and adolescents in sexual activities that they do not fully comprehend, are unable to give informed consent to and that violates the social taboos of family roles.

To this definition Tilman Furniss (1991) adds the rider: 'and which aim at the gratification of sexual demands and wishes of the abuser.'

Slightly amended, this definition was used by DHSS (1988) when issuing guidance on a multiagency basis. The more recent edition of *Working Together* (1991) has revised this advice and now uses the following definition: 'Actual or likely sexual exploitation of a child or adolescent. The child may be dependent and/or developmentally immature.'

These definitions are normative, highlighting the dependence of children and their inability to give informed consent. They do not refer to abuse only by a member of the child's household, although until 1988 it was more likely that the sexual abuse of a child or young person by a non-family member would be dealt with by the police working alone without resort to interagency child protection procedures. In these instances, it was regarded as a sexual assault and investigated through criminal procedures.

The distinction between sexual abuse and sexual assault is made on the basis of the relationship between the abuser and the child, although in fact all sexual abuse is also an assault. In sexual abuse, the sexual assault is perpetrated by a person who has responsibility for the child's wellbeing. That person could be a parent, stepparent, other family member (grandparent, sibling, etc), teacher, youth worker or baby-sitter. It is increasingly realised by professionals responsible for services to help sexually assaulted children, that especial harm is done where the assault is perpetrated by an adult in a position of trust and responsibility for the child. Whoever is identified as the abuser, it must be recognised that the child has been the victim of aggression in which sex is the primary weapon regardless of whether the incidents include actual physical violence or are perpetrated in a so-called 'loving' relationship. The identity of the abuser, as well as the reaction of the child's parent(s), will be crucial to the child's ability to describe the abuse and this must be borne in mind in any counselling situation.

It is also important to remember that:

1. victims may be either male or female, as could be the abuser,
2. the age of the child can range from any point from birth to adulthood, and
3. the range of sexual contact will be as wide as sexual knowledge and practice, for example: requiring the child to view adult sexual activity; fondling; digital penetration; oral sex; and penile penetration of both vagina and anus.

'He would pull his trousers and underpants down and grab hold of my hand and put it on his dick...' Eleven year old girl.

'He put a rude video on ... after the video had finished he took me up to the bathroom, told me to take my pants off and made me wee on his face...' Nine year old boy.

'One thing I have never done is kissed him, he's always wanted to but I wouldn't.' Fourteen year old girl after describing oral and vaginal sex.

The sexual acts may well also involve more than one person:

'I went with her and Dad was already in bed ... all three of us then stayed all night in the bed.'

The incident was part of an ongoing abusive relationship where 'Dad' was having sexual intercourse with his 14 year old stepdaughter and her friend.

These statements describing abuse illustrate the necessity to suspend belief about what may be 'normal' so that the actuality of the abuse incidents can be explored with the child in order to ascertain the extent of the trauma and, for the purposes of HIV/AIDS counselling, the risk at which the child may have been placed.

However, the typical scenario, particularly in intrafamilial abuse, is a progression from the less intimate forms of sexual activity, viewing 'soft porn' videos, showing similar magazines, exposure whether of whole body or genitals, and self-masturbation in front of the child.

Oral penetration may well be attempted quite early in this progression. Penile penetration of the anus and/or vagina usually comes after digital penetration, although ejaculation against the child's body and 'dry' intercourse may come at any stage.

Incidence

Up until 1988 the most reliable figures regarding the numbers of children who were alleging abuse, or suspected of being abused and needing protection, were to be found in the National Society for the Prevention of Cruelty to Children figures coming from their child protection registers. These registers covered nine per cent of the child population in England and Wales and, although, they may be criticised as unrepresentative in that they covered mainly Northern and Midland areas, they do provide one of the few reliable sources of long term information regarding identified abuse. These figures illustrate the increased recognition of sexual abuse after 1980. The exact numbers are masked by the fact that it was not until 1986, with the DHSS draft of the circular *Working Together*, that sexual abuse was officially recognised and defined as a register category. The national estimate for sexually abused children in 1986, using the criteria of registration, was 6,330 (Susan J Creighton 1988).

The Department of Health (DoH) have been collating figures since 1988, as shown in Table 2.5.1.

Table 2.5.1 DoH figures for child sexual abuse

	0-17 YEARS
1988	6,400
1989	6,600
1990	6,700
1991	5,900

Source: Department of Health Local
Authority Statistics

The figures in Table 2.5.1 show little increase over the four years and in 1989 and 1990 formed a steady 0.6 per 1,000 population under the age of 18 years. By 1991 this figure had dropped to 0.55 per 1,000 population under the age of 18 years.

This definition of the problem, while almost certainly underestimating the incidence of child sexual abuse, does give a picture of the number of cases being dealt with through registration procedures at any one time. These children are those most likely to have either alleged abuse or believed to be at risk of abuse because of their

behaviour and circumstances. They will also form that section of the
population which is judged most in need of protection because of their
vulnerability to reabuse. It could be that these children should be
specifically targeted for HIV/AIDS information counselling because
of this very vulnerability. The ethical considerations of this course are
discussed in greater detail in chapter 7.

For purposes of comparison, one of the more widely quoted
prevalence studies is that undertaken by Baker and Duncan (1988) as
part of a MORI Survey of a nationally representative sample. Twelve
per cent of female respondents and eight per cent of males reported
that they had been sexually abused before the age of 16 years. From
these figures, Baker and Duncan estimated that 4.5 million adults in
Great Britain were sexually abused as children and that, potentially,
1,117,000 children in the general population will be sexually abused by
the age of 15 years. Of these 1,117,000, only 143,000 will be abused
within the family leaving potentially 974,000 likely to be abused by a
non-family member. These figures are reinforced by estimates of
undetected abuse by convicted offenders who may detail up to 73
victims before their first conviction.

It should, however, be remembered that figures estimating the
incidence of child sexual abuse are likely to be an underestimation
while the figures from prevalence studies will be greatly influenced by
the definition used and the method of questioning. Almost certainly,
the incidence will be but the tip of the iceberg. Currently, there is no
reliable information as to the exact number. (For further details of this
problem *see* E. Vizard 1989.)

Recognition of abuse

Many victims may never reveal that they have been abused, or may not
talk about the incidents until they are adults. An understanding of the
process of uncovering abuse is not only an important element in any
assessment of the problem but also vital if victims are to receive
appropriate remedial help.

Understanding the barriers and difficulties which prevent children
from talking about abuse is necessary for both police and social
workers investigating abuse. This includes not only the physical and/
or verbal threats used to silence children but also the societally imposed
inhibitions to talking about sexual matters. HIV/AIDS counsellors
also need to appreciate these difficulties. They have to obtain clear and
explicit details of sexual activity in order to help the child and/or the
child's carers assess the risk of HIV infection, the need for counselling
and/or testing.

Much of the guidance refers to children and does not differentiate between the infant of five and the young person of 15 years when discussing, for example, interview procedures. Although it will be obvious when thought is given to the subject, it is not acknowledged that the restraints for a five year old are very different from the inhibitions to speech experienced by the older child. It is vital to bear in mind issues not only of gender, ethnic origin and religious background but also age and developmental perspectives when planning an interview or considering the relevance of information already uncovered.

Two primary modes of disclosure have been outlined in literature on the subject (*see* for example Sgroi 1982 and Sorenson and Snow 1991).

These are the disclosures revealed by chance — the so-called accidental disclosures — and those which are purposeful. The younger child is more likely to make an accidental disclosure, while the older, particularly adolescent, child is more likely to disclose purposely, and often in anger. Sanzier (1989), in a sample of 156 sexually abused children, found that over half (55 per cent) reports were purposeful.

On the other hand, in a sample of 116 cases where abuse had subsequently been validated by a conviction (94 per cent) and/or medical collaboration (6 per cent), 74 per cent of disclosures were accidental rather than purposeful. Further, and more alarming, 72 per cent of these victims denied being sexually abused when first approached about the possibility. The most common process was a movement from denial to tentative disclosure, followed by active disclosure where 96 per cent of the children were eventually able to give detailed first person accounts of the abuse. The process of tentative disclosure involves statements which minimise and distance the abuse, such as indicating it happened a long time ago, or that it only happened once. In fact, 66 per cent of these children were still being abused at the time they were making initial denials or tentative disclosures. (Sorenson and Snow 1991).

The interviewer needs also to understand the significance of each specific developmental stage with the limitations and advantages of each stage. A review of literature (e.g. Berliner 1983, Hindman 1987) appears to identify three specific stages — preschool, 5/6 to puberty, and postpubertal, although Berliner subdivides more fully, separating the 6 to 9/10 from the 9/10 to 12/13 age groups. These stages appear to fit comfortably with the well researched information available regarding cognitive development and the acquisition of moral and ethical concepts. (*See* section 1 for more detailed discussion).

Role of religion

No discussion of the development of children's sexual thinking or their attitudes to disclosing sexual activity can be complete without some discussion of the role of social and religious values. While there may have been a decline in attendance at church, there can be little doubt about the influence of Christian morality on attitudes to sexuality. The world depicted by 'The Secret World of Sex' is the world of many grandparents, if not parents. It underlies the blaming of women and ignorance of sexuality which was characteristic of English society as little as 40 years ago (Steve Humphries 1988). Religion and morality, particularly sexual morality, have long been interconnected, strongly influencing teaching about sexual matters. While some sex roles are biologically based, more are socially induced and reinforced by sex role stereotypes. These stereotypes are beginning to be acquired by children as young as two and are at their strongest at ages six and seven. They will influence what children are able to disclose, and how. They will also influence what adults are able to see and hear and how they interpret that material. Unfortunately, in both adults and children these factors make it harder, not easier, for children to disclose sexual abuse.

Margaret Kennedy (1992) gives a helpful account of the particular restraints on victims within the Christian community.

Validation of statements of abuse

Faced with all the difficulties many adults have in believing the actuality of sexual abuse to the real child (Summit 1988), the normal denial of most abusers and the apparent lack of collaborative evidence, it is often necessary to look at circumstantial evidence which indicates whether an allegation is valid or not.

This has two parts. One is the internal evidence held within the statement itself. The other is contained in other evidence found in the behaviour of the child, the history of the family, and the medical assessment. In an ideal world the evidence available would contain the following elements:

1. Spontaneous complaint by the child to a reliable adult such as a teacher;
2. Supporting circumstantial evidence by way of the behaviour of the child which is that associated with sexual abuse;
3. Investigative interview, on videotape, which confirms the spontaneous complaint and which is conducted according to evidentially sound principles;
4. Supporting medical evidence, either direct physical evidence or a history of somatic complaints which are associated with abuse;
5. Supporting forensic evidence such as semen on the child's clothing;

6. Evidence which indicated that the alleged abuser had opportunity to abuse the child;
7. Observation by sight or hearing by a third party of some part of the abuse — which may not necessarily have made sense at the time; and
8. Confession by the alleged abuser;
9. Family history.

Child's statement

> In general the interview is the heart of a sexual assault case. The better the statement, the better the case. In child sexual assault situations, the child's description of what happened is the most important — and often the only — evidence.
>
> (Berliner L. et al 1983.)

Research has been undertaken into the features which are most likely to be present in a reliable account of abuse. (Faler 1984; Jones and McGraw 1987; Wehrspann et al 1987.)

The most persuasive features include explicit detail, appropriate emotional affect and a story told in the first person from the child's point of view. Few children are able to give initial statements which contain all the details of the abuse. Statements which contain details of sights, sounds and smells which would be outside the child's experience had they not experienced sexual abuse will add great veracity to the account. However, single episodes of abuse, particularly if bizarre or traumatic, will be remembered in greater detail than episodes which are frequent and have occurred repeatedly over time. The coping mechanisms of a frequently abused child may lie in the child's ability to forget the details of the abuse. In these circumstances, the child may concentrate on a particular feature of the room which will be recalled more vividly than, for example, whether or not the abuser was wearing socks.

It is likely that the child who has been frequently abused will remember further details and may change aspects of the account. Changes in the account should not necessarily be equated with false allegations. They may be more believable than the child coached to make an allegation who sticks unwaveringly to the same, often undetailed story.

Threats, particularly of violence, may not be a feature of the initial disclosure but such threats are frequently uncovered at a later stage. The threats are not necessarily directly related to consequences of disclosure. In a violent household they do not need to be.

'My first ever memory is when I was 3 years old, I remember my Dad hitting me because I used to spit my food out.' Teenage incest victim recalling family life.

Nor should the power of threats against family pets be underestimated.

Mother explained that the cat was found squashed between Sharon's bed and the wall and there was no explanation for this, although the other children blame Sharon for the cat's death.

Common reactions associated with appropriate emotional affect are anxiety, fear, embarrassment, disgust and anger. A flat emotional response as if 'telling a story' has been associated with false allegations of abuse. On the other hand, it may also be associated with posttraumatic stress syndrome; it is then likely to be found in the child's reaction to other facets of life. It may also result from circumstances where the child has been required to repeat the account of abuse many times. In this situation it is advisable, if possible, to check the emotional status of the child when abuse was first alleged. It could also relate to the child's efforts to create distance from the overwhelming feelings associated with the abuse. This may be a feature where the child is also unable to recall precise details of the abuse.

Statements which are personal to the child and contain personal pronouns and name are more likely to be credible. The child is telling the story of what actually happened to them.

Medical and forensic evidence

While estimates of supporting medical evidence in sexually abused children vary, a figure of around 15 per cent of cases appears to be generally accepted (Kerns 1981, Paul 1977). Unequivocal medical and forensic evidence can be very helpful in that it is more likely to result in a confession and obviate the need for a child to appear in court. It also makes it extremely difficult for either the abuser or child or other members of the family to withdraw the allegation.

Medical evidence is sometimes confused with forensic evidence and consequently overemphasised. Medical evidence can only support the probability of abuse, and is but part of the supporting evidential assessment. The lack of medical evidence does not rule out abuse. Indeed, much sexual abuse of children would not lead to physical signs visible to examination. Even if there is medical evidence it cannot be used to positively identify the abuser. This is very different from forensic evidence which may positively identify the abuser. Even if there is medical evidence of abuse, it is still rare to also find forensic evidence positively identifying the abuser.

Family history

When the family history of a victim of abuse is examined, there is frequently a history of abuse in either or both parents and other family members. This is, of course, very different from implying that abuse victims will grow up either to be the parents of abused children or abusers. Many do not. But a background history of abuse seems to militate against parental ability to protect their own children, unless the parents have been able to deal effectively with the consequences of their own abuse. A family history of abuse does not identify the abuser of the child, although it may point to a range of possible suspects. It does appear to increase the probability that the child is making a valid allegation of abuse.

Witnesses

While it is uncommon for there to be a witness of the actual abuse, knowledge of its occurrence may be more general than is always discovered.

> Karen knew about John's abuse from the beginning and felt guilty that she did not stop it happening. She described listening to her brother cry as it was taking place.

This information came to light in therapy with the siblings only after their abusive father had left home. At the time, Karen was only asked whether her father had touched her. He had not, but she was too frightened of him, and felt too guilty about her brother, to volunteer the information that she had of her brother's abuse.

Information held by other family members may assume significance only when the victim makes an allegation. It may only come to light if work with the non-abusing parent and siblings is supportive and enabling, and they are asked about events in the household they could not understand or which now have a new significance.

This is especially true in multiple abuse situations where the involvement of peers in group activities is designed not only for the sexual gratification of the adults but also to further enmesh the children in collusive secrecy. A knowledge of group dynamics is vital to enabling witnesses/participants to talk about their own and others experiences.

Confession by the alleged abuser

The more convincing the evidence the more likely it is that there will be a confession. A premature exposure of suspicion of abuse gives the abuser time to find alternative and credible explanations. An allegation of sexual abuse is more often a crisis for the professional than for the child who has been living through the experience. Careful planning of the investigation to gather as much direct and circumstantial evidence as possible is essential and must be balanced against issues of immediate protection for the child. An unplanned hasty investigation may result in short term protection but is unlikely to result in long term safety.

Accommodation syndrome

One of the factors which reinforced popular belief that children lie about sexual abuse was the persistent tendency of children who mad statements about abuse, to withdraw these statements and state they had been mistaken. This was put into its proper perspective by Summit (1983) in his seminal paper *The Child Sexual Abuse Accommodation Syndrome.*

Child sexual abuse is commonly described as a syndrome of secrecy and helplessness into which the child is entrapped by the adult abuser. To survive emotionally, the child must accommodate the abuse by adapting their own behaviour to make sense of that of the all powerful adult. It should be remembered that much sexual abuse will start at a young age when children are still developmentally dependent on adults. In 1979 in the US, for example, the average age abused children were initiated into abusive activities was nine years. In England in 1990 10 per cent of boys registered and 21 per cent of girls in the five to eight year age range were placed on Child Protection Registers in need of protection from sexual abuse.

The behaviour patterns which adult common sense dictates should be expected from children in the face of violation do not occur. Children do not rush for help but keep quiet although their behaviour may sometimes allow sensitive adults to guess what is happening.

When the child eventually discloses purposefully, the disclosure may be conflicting and unconvincing. Typically this will be an angry teenager who has already been labelled a delinquent, who is reacting against adult authority.

> 'The community policeman would not believe me (social worker) let alone Mary when she began to disclose abuse and the name of the abuser.' Comment by a social worker regarding a 13 year old who had a six year history of stealing and behaviour problems.

At this point, and without sympathetic adult support, faced with the reaction the child has been taught to expect — denial, disbelief and anger — the child will retract. If there is already a history of acting out, antisocial behaviour and/or promiscuity and particularly if the parents are respectable and well spoken, it will not be difficult for many to believe the retraction, not the original allegation.

Sorenson and Snow (1991) found that 22 per cent of their sample retracted their statements of abuse. The reasons to recant which were given are:

1. Pressure from perpetrator;
2. Pressure from family;
3. Negative personal consequences;
4. Videotaping;
5. Retelling parents;
6. Judicial proceedings;
7. Investigatory police or CPS

Ninety three per cent of these did go on to reaffirm their allegation. Retraction should, perhaps, be seen as part of the normal process when children embark on the almost impossible task of explaining to adults about the sexual use other adults have made of their bodies.

Summary

- Outline of the difficulties inherent in finding a satisfactory definition.

- Incidence and prevalence, distinguishing these concepts; and

- Attempting an estimate of the size of the problem.

- Some of the barriers which prevent children disclosing abuse.

- Guidance as to how the validity of individual disclosures may be assessed.

- Brief explanation of why some abused children may subsequently retract their statements.

References and bibliography

Baker A W and Duncan S P, 1985 Child sexual abuse: a study of prevalence in Great Britain. *Child Abuse and Neglect* **9**: 457-67. Pergamon Press Ltd.

Berliner L, et al, 1983 *Child Sexual Abuse Investigation: A Curriculum for Training Law Enforcement Officers in Washington State,* Criminal Justice Training Commission, Victims of Sexual Assault Programs, Department of Social and Health Services, State of Washington, 19-24.

Creighton S J, 1984 *Trends in Child Abuse.* NSPCC.

Creighton S J, 1988 Incidence of Child Abuse and Neglect in *Early Prediction and Prevention of Child Abuse* Ed Browne K, Davis C and Stratton P. John Wiley and Sons, Chichester, New York.

DHSS and Welsh Office, 1988 *Working Together — A Guide to Arrangements for Inter-Agency Co-operation for the Protection of Children from Abuse.* HMSO — revised 1991 under the auspices of the Home Office, Department of Health, Department of Education and Science and Home Office *Working Together under the Children Act 1989 — A Guide to Arrangement for Inter-Agency Co-operation for the Protection of Children from Abuse.* HMSO.

Department of Health *Personal social services local authority statistics. Children and young persons on child protection registers* years ending 31 March 1988, 1989, 1990, 1991. England. HMSO.

Faller C K, 1984 Is the child victim of sexual abuse telling the truth. In *Child Abuse and Neglect* **8**: 473-81.

Furniss Tilman, 1991 *The multiprofessional handbook of child sexual abuse: integrated management, therapy and legal intervention.* Routledge, London and New York.

Hindman J, 1987 *Step by step — sixteen steps towards legally sound sexual abuse investigations.* Alexandria Associates, Ontario.

Humphries S, 1988 *A secret world of sex. Forbidden fruit. The British experience 1900–1950.* Sedgwick and Jackson.

Jones D P H and McGraw, J M, 1987 Reliable and fictitious accounts of sexual abuse to children. *Journal of Interpersonal Violence* **2** (1) March 1987: 27-45.

Kennedy M, 1992 Christianity — help or hindrance for the abused child or adult. *Child Abuse Review* **5** (3): 3-6.

Kerns D L, 1981 Medical assessment in child sexual abuse. In Mrazek

P B and Kempe C H (eds) *Sexually abused children and their families* pp126–41. Pergamon.

Paul D M, 1977 The medical examination in sexual offences against children. *Medicine, Science and the Law* **17**: 251–58.

Sanzier M, 1989 Disclosures of child sexual abuse. *Psychiatric Clinics of North America* **12**.

Schetchter M D and Roberge L, 1976 Sexual exploitation. In Helfer R E and Kempe C H (eds) *Child abuse and neglect: the family and the community.* Ballinger, Cambridge, Mass.

Sgroi S, Blick L and Porter F, 1982 A conceptual framework for child sexual abuse. In Sgroi S (ed) *Handbook of clinical intervention in child sexual abuse.* Lexington Books.

Sorenson T and Snow B, 1991 How children tell: the process of disclosure in child sexual abuse. *Child Welfare* **LXX** (1) Jan-Feb 1991: 3–15.

Summit R C, 1983 The child sexual abuse accommodation syndrome. *Child abuse and neglect.* **7**: 177-93.

Summit R C, 1988 Hidden victims, hidden pain. Societal avoidance of child sexual abuse. In Wyatt G E and Powell G J (eds) *The lasting effects of child sexual abuse.* Sage Publications Inc.

Vizard E, 1989 Incidence and prevalence of child sexual abuse. *The consequences of child sexual abuse association for child psychology and psychiatry.* Occasional Papers No 3, Series Ed Dr J Ouston.

Wehrspann W H, Steinhauer P D, Krajner-Diamond H, 1987 Criteria and methodology for assessing credibility of sexual abuse allegation. *Canadian Journal of Psychiatry* **32** Oct 1987: 615–23.

6 Investigation

Introduction

Working Together 1988 and 1991 have laid the foundations for inter-agency responses to child sexual abuse. There will be individual differences in service response and coordination in different areas of the country which will not exactly follow *Working Together.* However, the broad structure, encouraging co-operation between agencies with honest communication and information sharing, should now be a common pattern.

The model for investigation outlined in this chapter is based on the interagency model as recommended in *Working Together.* It assumes not only an interagency trust in exchange of information but also a planned response which takes the time-scale of the child into account.

It includes the involvement of children and their parents in the process but aims to be primarily child-centred, maximising the potential for the abused child to talk about the abuse, while minimising the trauma of multiple investigative interviews and medical examinations.

It is based on the assumption that the responsibility for the abuse rests with the abuser not the child, nor the non-abusing parent. While this may appear axiomatic, it is still not infrequent to hear the partner of the abuser being blamed for being non-protective and, even if overt blame of the victim is no longer as common, it still occurs.

'Once the stepfather became a member of the household, he was faced with Claire's obsessive interest in sex... Many children go through such a phase... Unfortunately, in this case, Claire's sexual interest reached a degree which should perhaps be called pathological.' Stepfather's therapist describing the behaviour of a nine year old.

'Mother was abused herself as a child so she should have recognised the signs in her daughter.' Comment made in an Initial Child Protection Conference.

The investigative model initially aims at removing the abuser rather than the child. This process, of necessity, must incorporate work to strengthen the protective ability of the non-abusing carer. Overall, the aim is to prevent further abuse and reduce emotional trauma to the child, including the secondary abuse of the investigative process, to a minimum.

This is the ideal but, in reality, the process is frequently at best barely good enough and distressingly frequently a failure.

'The second part deals with some of the numerous practical problems which always ensure that the intervention never works as it should according to the clever theory of the first part. The second part addresses some of the countless obstacles for helping sexually abused children and their families which makes me jubilant if I do not get nine out of ten but only eight out of ten cases wrong.'

Thus Tilman Furniss introduces his work based on many years of skilled intervention with sexually abusing families (Furniss T 1991). Only rarely does a case sit neatly into a clear theoretical model, while only too often does it start wrongly at referral and go from bad to worse. It is relatively easy to quote what appears to be good and recommended practice at the present time but:

'at present the half-blind are talking to the blind. One of the major causes of secondary damage to sexually abused children and of burn-out in professionals is the immense pressure on professionals and the feeling that we have to pretend we can see fully and that we know well how to act. But none of us does yet.'

(Furniss T 1991.)

The guidance in this chapter, indeed, in the whole book should be read with this in mind.

Recognition of abuse

Signs and symptoms of sexual abuse are discussed and put into a developmental perspective in section 1.

The barriers to recognition and discussion of abuse are discussed in section 2, chapter 8.

However, it cannot be emphasised too often that many of the signs and symptoms associated with sexual abuse are also associated with other problems. It is important to look at the aetiology of each symptom and weigh the evidence for alternative explanations. In the absence of direct allegation or admission, it is only when there is no alternative explanation for the signs and symptoms, or many of them, that sexual abuse should be considered as the most likely explanation. Too often the conclusion that the child has been sexually abused is jumped upon with only flimsy signs and without examining alternative explanations. A correct diagnosis of abuse is different from an identification of the abuser. Protection of the child demands an open mind and an ability to explore all possibilities.

While validity through research has been established for sexually specific symptoms such as compulsive masturbation, over-sexualised behaviour and a knowledge of sexual activity which is well in advance of that expected of a similar aged child at a similar developmental level, each of these symptoms may be influenced by 'observer bias' and needs to be evaluated carefully against objective data.

Referral to appropriate agency

While some children may disclose abuse unwittingly and others may disclose in anger, many children will be unable to discuss abusive experiences unless they feel safe to do so. In child sexual abuse, protection must come before therapy. The appropriate agency for referral for investigation will be a Social Services Department, or the NSPCC, or the Police because these three agencies have the authority to take protective action as well as the necessary investigative skills and training — see Figure 2.6.1.

It may be that in the course of the investigation an interview with the child or other family members will need to be organised with the help of a specialist worker, such as a child psychiatrist or psychologist, but this will be part of the planned process of investigating. Initial referral should not be made to Child Guidance or other agency without informing and involving the statutory protection agencies. Protection will be secured preferably by ensuring the alleged abuser leaves the household, but it may be necessary to remove the child.

Investigation

In the last five years the trend in investigation procedures has been towards closer liaison and planning between Social Services Departments and the Police. Even if the entire investigation is not planned on a joint basis, there will be considerable overlap in response. Even if the response is still on a separate agency basis, usually there will be some communication. (Jo Moran Ellis et al 1991.)

The advantages and disadvantages of joint investigation were being

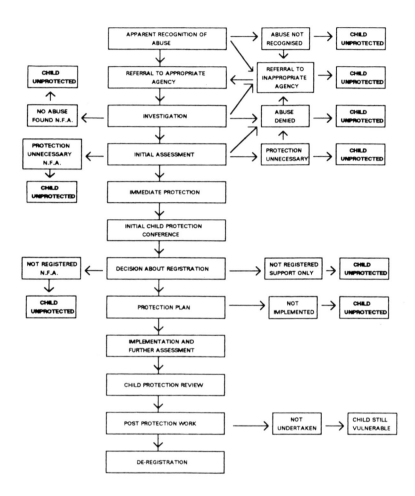

Figure 2.2.1.   Stages of process or: 'It is only too easy to leave an abused child unprotected'

discussed in the early eighties (*see*, for example, NSPCC 1984). Attention was drawn to the possible advantages of cooperation between Social Services and the Police by the Bexley Experiment. This has been seen as pioneering joint investigation although, in reality, it marked progress in joint understanding of the roles and responsibilities of each agency as a result of joint training, leading to cooperation in interviewing the child, rather than a joint investigation. It is now more common than not for the interview of the child victim to be undertaken jointly by police and social services personnel. It is still uncommon for this to be the case for the interview of the alleged perpetrator (Jo Moran Ellis et al 1991.)

Ideally, no investigation into an allegation of child sexual abuse will occur without preinvestigative planning between police and social services. Whether this planning is by telephone or by face-to-face meeting will depend on the speed of response needed and the geographical area.

There will be some circumstances when the response will need to be urgent. These include situations when the child is making a direct allegation and is asking for immediate help, or needs urgent medical assistance. They may also include situations where the gathering of forensic evidence is likely because there is, allegedly, a recent sexual act; where the alleged perpetrator is felt likely to take steps to silence the child; or where there is a real risk of harm to the child through self harm or running away.

In some rural areas, sheer distance may make regular face-to-face meetings organisationally difficult.

Whenever time permits and particularly when there is no direct allegation, a pre-investigative planning meeting should be held to decide the most appropriate response and plan the timescale. While this meeting will primarily involve police and social workers, it may also involve the doctor who will undertake any medical examination considered necessary, and the person who has details of the complaint or has amassed information amounting to serious suspicion of abuse. In many instances this could be a teacher or a psychiatrist/ psychologist who had been involved with the child for some time previously because there have been behavioural concerns. It is possible that the meeting could include the parent when it is that parent who has reason to believe that their child has been abused.

The meeting will consider all available evidence — behavioural signs, medical indications, circumstantial evidence and statements of the child in order to plan the investigation.

The best interest of the child should be the paramount consideration and should influence all decision-making. In addition, consideration must be given to informing the child's parents, if not already done, that abuse is suspected.

It may be necessary to initiate monitoring to gather more information at this stage. Alternatively, it may be felt that the next step is to interview the child.

Interviewing

In much official advice there appears to be lack of differentiation about the type and purpose of interviews with children where sexual abuse is suspected. The *Report of the Inquiry into Child Abuse in Cleveland* 1987 has led to the discrediting of the term 'disclosure interview'.

Dr Jones said:

> a fundamental problem of the 'disclosure' approach is that it is inherent in the concept that there is something to disclose. The problem is highlighted by those professionals who consider that the child is either disclosing or 'in denial'. The third and crucial alternative possibility, namely that the child has no sexual abuse to disclose, is not considered as a viable option ... it is important to remember that there are at least three possible situations:

> 1. The abuse has occurred and the child is speaking of it
> 2. The abuse has occurred and the child is unable to speak of it or is denying it
> 3. The ause has not occurred and the child cannot speak of it.
>
> (Cleveland Report 1987)

Unfortunately, and as outlined in the previous chapter, the occasions when the abused child does not choose to tell may be more frequent than many people would find it comfortable to believe.

Foresaking the term 'disclosure' interview has left terminological problems for the nomenclature of an interview at this stage. It is possibly more properly called an investigative interview. Whichever term is used, the danger is always that in trying to discover what has happened to the child, and whether it is abuse which necessitates taking protective action, an exaggerated sense of urgency can lead to inappropriate and leading questions. At its worse, such an interview is both traumatic and counterproductive. At best, and following such clearly laid out guidelines as those produced by Yuille (1988) and Hindman (1987), the interview will allow the child to talk about abuse, if it has happened, in a way which will be valid for use in court proceedings as necessary.

This interview is likely to be videotaped and should normally be undertaken jointly by the police and social services working together. While it may be helpful for the child to have the presence of a trusted adult in the room or behind a screen, it is not often advisable for a parent to be present. Children frequently feel guilty about the sexual contact and may well have been told their parent will be angry with them, or will not believe them. The presence of the parent in these circumstances is not helpful.

At least one of the interviewers should have training in interview techniques and an aptitude for working with children. Consideration must be given to the gender of the interviewers and whether the child has expressed a preference. Consideration must also be given to whether the child has communication problems such as hearing impairment or learning difficulties which point to a need for a specialist, who knows and understands the child, being present to help. The child may not be a first language English speaker or may come from an ethnic minority where social values and customs will need to be understood to conduct a satisfactory interview.

Above all, the interviewers will need to keep an open mind in order to respond to facts as they emerge without prejudice.

In summary those arranging the interview of the child must consider:

1. Age and gender of the child;
2. Developmental status of the child;
3. Ethnic origin and religious background of the child;
4. Whether there may be communication difficulties by reason of language or handicap;
5. Gender of the interviewer(s);
6. Presence or not of a trusted adult or parent.

Other interviews

Apart from the initial investigative interview, there may be need to conduct other interviews with the child. These should be kept to a minimum and should not be confused with interviews which form part of the therapeutic treatment plan for the child. Ongoing treatment may well reveal extra information which may, or may not, confirm the original allegation. The use of treatment to try to secure information to validate the allegation or suspicion that abuse has taken place is not only frequently counter-productive but also abusive in itself. Such material is unlikely to be available to use in a criminal investigation and is more likely to be challenged as therapist influenced in other proceedings. Therapeutic interviews have the purpose of helping the child make sense of events with the aim of helping to heal the hurt. To confuse this with the need to obtain evidence is unlikely to help the child overcome the abusive experience.

It may, however, be helpful to have a validating interview after the initial investigative interview. This would be held to increase understanding of, and to test the reliability of, the original allegation. It will be particularly helpful in situations where the allegation was made in the course of a custody dispute between the parents. In these circumstances, the child should be seen with the parent confirming the allegation. Careful note should be made of attempts by the parent to speak for the child, prompt or lead what the child is saying, or in other ways influence the content of the child's story. While research (D Jones 1988) indicates that even in the course of custody disputes, the incidence of false allegation is low, it is in this situation that it is believed that false allegations are more likely.

Validation of the interviews themselves is addressed in chapter 5.

Initial assessment

The initial assessment will address the areas of whether or not it appears likely that the abuse has occurred, whether the abuse is ongoing and where the child may best be placed in safety from further abuse while the investigation is completed.

It is obviously important that the alleged victim (and siblings) are protected from further abuse but the way this is done must take into account the emotional damage which can result from premature or inappropriate removal from known and loved carers.

The investigators should explain to the child the process of investigations and discuss the available options. The wishes and feelings of the child must be carefully listened to. In the last resort, adults have responsibility for ensuring the safety of children and must take responsibility for doing so — whilst explaining to the child the reasons for their decisions.

Immediate protection

The initial assessment will look at the protective ability of the non-abusing carer and the willingness of the alleged abuser to stay away from the victim throughout the investigation. While it has always been possible to find ways of helping the alleged abuser leave the home, this as a preferred method was highlighted by the Cleveland Report and is enshrined in the guidance issued with the *Children Act 1989* — in particular *Working Together* 1991.

There will be some occasions when it is clear that either both carers were involved with the abuse, or one carer, while not involved is nevertheless unable to accept the possibility that abuse could have happened. In these circumstances, the child should be placed with a family member or trusted adult who is able to support the child through the trauma of the investigation. This option may also be closed, in which case the child may have to be placed with foster parents. At this stage is is preferable not to place an abused child with other children who also may have been abused. It takes some time to discover the full vulnerability of each individual child, as well as the range of behavioural problems resulting from their abusive experiences.

Some abused children will already have started involving younger children in sexual activities which are abusive. This may be more common in the teenage group but instances have been found in quite young (six and seven year old) children. Victims are also more vulnerable to such involvement with other children replicating and reinforcing their victim status.

In the first instance placements will be negotiated by voluntary agreement. Parents should be encouraged to exercise their responsibility for their child's welfare in a constructive way. The social worker should try to work in partnership with the parents and in consultation with the child, provided that this approach does not jeopardise the welfare of the child. The aim is to try to provide protection for the child without needing to resort to emergency court action or care proceedings.

When accommodation is provided for the child outside the child's home, this should be done by written agreement with the parents. This agreement will reflect the fact that the parents retain parental responsibility but are either unwilling or unable to provide protection for their child at that time.

In coming to any such voluntary arrangement, the social worker will need to keep in mind the following checklist:

1. Child's needs;

2. Parent's capacity to understand and provide for their child's needs;

3. Parent's ability to keep to the agreed plan;

4. Wishes of the child — always remembering to take into account the child's age and understanding of the situation;

5. Type of placement best suited to the child's needs; and

6. Contact arrangements between the child and the child's parents, particularly if one or more carer is the alleged abuser.

Such negotiations in the face of an allegation of sexual abuse, particularly when it is denied, are difficult. It is hoped that by making the attempt there will be a reduction in the number of children removed from home in an emergency without careful regard to the alternatives. This has, in the past, added to the child's feelings of guilt. Unfortunately, and on the other hand, removing the alleged abuser can also result in scapegoating the child left in the family.

A young adult was discussing her feelings at the time she had alleged sexual abuse when aged 13 years. She was asked whether the decision to exclude her father (the abuser) from the home, rather than remove her to care, had been the most helpful decision for her. She thought carefully and replied:

> 'There was no way you could have made the right choice. I would have hated being removed from home, but I felt very guilty that my father was not there and my mother and sister kept telling me it was my fault and that I should have kept quiet.'

Perhaps it should be recognised more often that when there is an allegation of sexual abuse, there is no right way forward. With luck (and skill) we will only be able to provide, at best, the least bad of the inadequate alternatives available.

When it is impossible or unsafe for the child to negotiate a voluntary arrangement with the carers, the child must be protected using an Emergency Protection Order and/or Care Proceedings.

Multiple abuse and extra familial abuse

The discussion so far has centred on situations where the alleged abuse is believed to have taken place within the family situation.

In reality, sexual abuse occurs in a wide variety of situations and the response will need to be tailored to the specifics of each situation. Abuse outside the family may occur when the child is one of many abused children and where there are many abusers. This is especially complicated when the abusers are believed to be family members as well as adults from outside the family — as was alleged both in Rochdale and the Orkneys.

The alleged abuser may be in a position of trust and authority such as a teacher or youth leader. Alternatively, the alleged abuser may be a family friend or a baby-sitter. It is rarer, but not unknown, for the abuser to be a complete stranger to the child. Many paedophiles will either choose occupations or ways of life which bring them into contact with the children, or will cultivate friendships with families which contain children.

One of the results of work with paedophiles and child molesters has been an increase in knowledge about the way in which they operate. It has destroyed many myths.

Child molester talks to parents

Who am I?

I am not the mythical 'dirty old man' who hangs about in the bushes outside school.

I am probably well known and liked by your child and you.

I can be a man or a woman.

I can be a child older than yours.

I can be of any race, hold any religious belief and have any sexual preference.

I can be a parent, a stepparent, other relative, family friend, teacher, clergyman, baby-sitter or anyone who works with children.

I am most likely a stable, employed respected member of the community.

My education and intelligence don't prevent me from molesting your child.

I am a person who has access to your child, and I will do things to gain your child's trust.

I can be anybody.

(Center for Behavioural Intervention 1991)

There must be sufficient flexibility in the investigative process to accomodate all these situations. Broadly, the differences are found in three main variables. These are: whether the alleged abuser has care of the child, i.e. a parent, stepparent, foster parent, residential care worker; whether the abuse situation involves a number of abusers and/or a number of non-related children and finally, whether the alleged abuser is known to the child and family, or is a stranger. Investigation in all instances will need to be planned. The differences are to be found in the issues surrounding protection, the scale of the operation, and number of personnel to be involved. At this point in time, the spectre of HIV/AIDS is more likely to be raised in situations of multiple abuse involving strangers but, with the spread of infection to all sections of society, it must always be considered as a possibility in planning treatment.

There will also be an adaptation of the process of investigations to take into account the situation of allegations against professionals working with children and foster parents or residential workers. With regard to professionals working with children, care should be taken that the investigatory process is in line with established disciplinary proceedings. While the allegation may not be sustainable in criminal proceedings, it may well be felt unsafe to allow the person concerned to continue in employment in contact with children. It would be a further abuse of the child if the process of investigation had to be repeated to fit existing disciplinary processes.

In addition careful thought will need to be given to the disposition of records of any such investigations, balancing natural justice and the rights of the individual against the need to protect children. The events which led to the dismissal of the Director of Social Services in

Calderdale (Roycroft B, et al 1989), as well as the enquiry held in East Sussex (East Sussex County Council 1988) regarding a music teacher, illustrate how vital it is to keep at least some record of complaints about individuals. The report of the enquiry held after the conviction of a head teacher in Cornwall (Cornwall County Council 1987) provides other insights into the difficult area of gathering evidence of suspicion about such individuals.

Foster parents pose different problems in that they are one group particularly vulnerable to false allegations, and because they also have 24 hour care of the child. Any investigation of abuse allegedly by a foster parent must include careful thought as to whether the allegation had been triggered by an incident related to post traumatic stress syndrome. The planning which results from receiving an allegation must balance the trauma of immediate removal of children in the household against the risks of abuse.

Medical examinations

In all cases where sexual abuse is alleged, consideration must be given to whether a medical examination will be required. This should be part of the initial planning between the police, social services and the health service.

The police may wish for a medical investigation because it is thought to be the only way to collect collaborative evidence. Social workers may see a medical examination as a low priority to be undertaken as part of the treatment process.

For many the medical examination will still have connotations of abuse and invasion of privacy. The myth remains that the examining doctor will only be interested in the child's genital area and that the examination can, in itself, be abusive.

In reality the examination must take into account the need for forensic investigation and the collection of evidence. However, the assessment and treatment of any medical complications and the needs of the child and the child's parents for support and counselling will take priority.

The child should not be subjected to multiple medical examinations, and be made to feel as comfortable as possible throughout by careful attention to timing and setting. They should be accompanied by an adult of their choice whom they find supportive. It is important that they are consulted about the gender of the examining doctor. While this is important for all children, it is particularly important for older children. However, while adults may assume that, for example, a child would prefer to be examined by a doctor of the same gender, one must not forget the strict sex role stereotyping of six and seven year olds. It is not infrequent for children of this age to say to the examining doctor: 'You can't be a doctor, you're a lady!'.

In order to avoid the necessity of the child repeating allegations, the examining doctor should be given full details of the joint interview of the child. A medical history is also helpful, although this may be obtainable as part of the examination.

The consent of the parent will be necessary for medical examination unless the court has ruled otherwise. The child also needs to understand the reasons for the examination and give consent to cooperate. (This issue is examined in more detail in Chapter 8.)

Many children will have fantasies (which may in fact be reality) about bodily damage as the result of the abuse. All victims of sexual abuse should be offered the opportunity of medical examination whether or not it is necessary for evidential purposes. A follow-up examination separate from the investigation process should also be considered.

Any medical examination of a child where abuse is alleged should include a thorough assessment of the whole child. This will include measurement of height and weight as well as examination of eyes, ears, mouth and main body system. Examination of the genital area should always come after these primary examinations and at a time the child feels at ease with the examining doctor.

It may be that the subject of HIV/AIDS infection will be raised by the child or parents during this initial investigation, or the subject may be raised at a later stage. It is important that the examining doctor has an understanding of area resources for pre-test counselling and an established, easily accessible route for referral.

Initial child protection conference

Child Protection Conferences are regarded as central to the effective interagency management of child protection. The administrative processes of convening conferences are undertaken by social services departments who, for most areas, convene, provide the administrative support and the chairs for the conferences.

The conference will act as a forum for exchange of information and formulation of interagency plans for assessment, treatment and protection of the child. Attendance at the conference will be limited to those who have a contribution to make and a 'need to know'. The parents of the child as well as the child may well attend part, if not all, of the conference.

The conference is not a legal forum in which to decide who is responsible for abusing the child. Indeed contributions to the conference are not admissible in criminal proceedings. It is concerned with creating the conditions for a thorough multi-disciplinary assessment of what has gone wrong so that it is possible to provide both protection and remedial help for the child.

Contributions are confidential to the conference. Care should be taken that neither records of the conference nor information exchanged therein are made available on other than a 'need to know' basis. Each professional should try to make an opportunity to discuss their individual contribution separately with the family and/or the child.

Each agency subscribing to the child protection procedures should have guidance for the preservation of confidentiality. Destruction of information obtained from the proceedings once it is no longer needed to protect or help the child should also be prescribed in procedures.

Summary

- Investigation of abuse.
- Initial recognition.
- Initial Child Protection Conferences.
- Difficulties in interviewing children; and
- Preserving confidentiality.

References and bibliography

A child molester talks to parents 1991. A brochure developed under the auspices of the Center for Behavioural Intervention, Beaverton, Oregon, USA.

Butler-Sloss E, 1988 *Report of the inquiry into child abuse in Cleveland 1987.* HMSO.

Children Act 1989 — in particular, Guidance and Regulations Vol. 1 — Court Orders.

Cornwall County Council, 1987 *Child abuse in schools.* Internal report.

DHSS and Welsh Office, 1988 *Working Together — A Guide to Arrangements for Inter-Agency Cooperation for the Protection of Children from Abuse.* HMSO — revised 1991 under the auspices of the Home Office, Department of Health, Department of Education and Science and Home Office *Working Together under the Children Act 1989 — A Guide to Arrangements for Inter-Agency Cooperation for the Protection of Children from Abuse.* HMSO.

East Sussex County Council, 1988 *Review of disciplinary procedures and other matters.* Internal Report.

Furniss Tilman, 1991 *The multiprofessional handbook of child sexual abuse: integrated management, therapy and legal intervention.* Routledge, London and New York.

Hindman J, 1987 *Step by step — sixteen steps towards legally sound sexual abuse investigations.* Alexandria Associates, Ontario.

Jones D and Seig A, 1988 Child Sexual Abuse in Custody or Visitation Cases. A report of 20 cases in Nicholson E G and Bulkley J (eds) *Sexual abuse allegations in custody and visitation cases: a resource book for judges and court personnel.* pp.22–36. America Bar Association, Washington DC.

Moran-Ellis J, Conroy S, Fielding N, Tunstill J, 1991 *Investigation of child sexual abuse — an executive summary 1991.* Department of Sociology, University of Surrey, Guildford.

NSPCC S.W. Working Party, 1984 *Developing a child centred response to sexual abuse.* A discussion paper. Nov. 1984, NSPCC.

Roycroft B, Miles B, Philp D, 1989 *Calderdale social services inquiry.* Metropolitan Borough of Calderdale.

Yuille J C, 1988 The systematic assessment of children's testimony. *Canadian Psychology* **29**(3): 247–62.

7 Post investigation

It would be impossible in this context to do justice to the many and varied approaches to helping and supporting sexually abused children and their families. Indeed, although there is a paucity of research into outcome related to therapy, there is some indication that the method chosen is less important than the skills of the therapist undertaking the work. (Luborsky et al 1986.)

Instead a method of assessment, looking at both protection and therapy needs, is outlined, with brief discussion regarding the advantages of different therapeutic interventions. This outline emphasises the role of the non-abusing carer as the single most important therapeutic and protective factor for the child. It also discusses the conflict between the desire of family members to be reunited and the real risk of reabuse this course may involve.

Assessment and treatment

Three elements will need to be considered both in terms of protection and damage to the child. These elements concern the characteristics of the adult(s) who has used the child victim for their own sexual gratification; the child victim; and the environment, including protective adults, which surrounds the child victim.

Each of these elements interlock and will dictate the measures necessary for the child to be protected, and the intervention necessary to repair the harm of the abuse. This intervention may include therapy with the abuser so that contact between the child and the abuser is possible.

Alleged abuser

Characteristics of abuse:
Relationship with child

Carer/parent
Family friend/relation
Professional
Stranger

Length and number of assault episodes	Long-term/repeated/regular
	Long-term/occasional
	Short-term/repeated
	Single episodes
Type of assault	'Loving'
	Verbal threats
	Physical violence/threats
	Bribes/enticement
Responsibility/denial	Total denial
	Accept act not responsibility
	Accept act and responsibility
	Accepts risk of self to children

Protection issues

In the initial stage of investigation, the alleged abuser should not have contact with the victim of abuse. Clearly this is more easily achieved if the abuser is not a member of the child's household. Issues of protection, not only of the victim but also other children who may be, or become, targets for the abuser, must be considered. Where there is knowledge of long-term abuse or more than one victim, particularly when violence is involved, the matter should be placed before the court quickly and protection addressed through custody or bail conditions. Statements by the abuser that this was a one-off unplanned episode should be viewed with scepticism. It is unusual for an abuser to be ascertained on the occasion of their first offence. It may, however, be the first offence against any one particular victim. At the assessment stage, no assumptions should be made that the abuser is only a risk to either children in the family, or non-family members. Neither should it be assumed that the offences are gender specific. While acceptance of responsibility may provide a hopeful prognosis for help, it should not be an excuse for not separating offender from victim in these early stages.

Therapy issues

The reaction of the abusers will range from total denial to an acceptance that they are a risk to children. The latter will be a less common reaction. In one survey of 41 families where sexual abuse was alleged, only six abusers accepted any degree of responsibility in the initial stages of the investigation.

The denial can start as total denial of both abuse and responsibility. This may be followed by an acknowledgement that the child might have been abused but that the abuser must be someone else. There are interesting but unvalidated indications that the reaction of parents to the information that their child has been abused, may give an indication of the abuser. Those parents who leap immediately to the conclusion that they are being accused are more likely to be responsible than those who address the needs of the child and speculate as to who could be responsible (Wills D, 1983).

From this stance the next stage is to accept the act but proffer excuses which disclaim responsibility.

> 'If she says I did it I must have done but I don't remember.'
> 'I was drunk at the time.'
> 'I was only teaching him...'
> 'She led me on...'
> 'She looks just like her mother...'
> 'I woke up and found him in bed masturbating me...'

These sorts of justifications are the most common stage for the abuser who accepts the abuse but has yet to accept responsibility.

Denial may also be of the act as an action of a sexual nature; the act as a planned event; and the act as part of a pattern of fantasies and past offences. These denials may also be shared by professionals working with families where there is abuse. Thus statements such as:

> 'there are indications that the act was not of an aggressive nature and was probably committed in a "twilight state"... and that his inhibitions were probably not as high as they normally are.' Extract from an assessment report of an abuser.

have been used in reports to justify or minimise those actions. There appears to be little realisation that abusers who disown their actions in this way are actually more dangerous because they cannot take responsibility for ensuring it does not happen again.

Abusers will try to disarm the professional responsible for assessing their dangerousness in a number of ways. One is by way of 'religious conversion'. This usually takes the form of:

> Yes, I did abuse Mary but that was before I started going to Church. Now I know how wrong it was and I will never do it again so you don't have to worry and I don't have to have any other help.

An answer to this is to suggest that actions speak louder than words, and that since God only helps those who help themselves, the abuser may like to enlist God's help and support through the therapy programme.

Another is by way of emotionality, weeping, suicidal threats, and displays of great grief designed to gain sympathy while deflecting the assessor from issues of the abuse. In these circumstances, it is helpful to temporarily suspend the interview suggesting that it is only possible to address issues of responsibility with the adult side of the abuser. The interview recommences when the abuser is able to allow the adult side to regain control of the childish side so overcome with emotion.

Abusers may also use their own victimisation both to sidetrack the assessor and as an excuse for their behaviour. It should be made clear that discussion of abusive behaviour must be undertaken before regard is given to the victim status of the abuser. However, in a therapy situation, the victimisation may give helpful insights into the origin of the abusive fantasies and actions of the abuser. It will then need to be addressed in this setting.

While work with abusers will not normally form part of the work of HIV/AIDS counsellors, it is by understanding some of the denial processes that they may be more aware of the difficulties of victims and the complexities of unravelling what has actually happened between victim and abuser.

There are useful techniques which can be employed to minimise denial. It is more difficult to practise denial in situations when there is positive rapport. For this reason, time should be spent establishing such rapport, possibly through gathering a background social history, before the sexual abuse is discussed. It is helpful to read witness statements prior to the interview with the abuser so that distortions and minimisations can be picked up through a knowledge of what has already been alleged.

It is unhelpful to have the partner of the abuser present. Not only may this make it more difficult to admit to specific sexual acts but it also makes it more difficult to later retract a denial. There may be implicit or explicit threats to the continuation of the partnership:

> I am willing to stay with him because he only fondled her. I wouldn't stay if there had been penetration.

or more commonly:

> I don't believe it happened. If it did we couldn't stay together.

Denial may be a defence against anxiety. At each stage, there should be a clear explanation of the purpose of the assessment and an active encouragement of questions in an effort to keep anxiety to a minimum.

Assessment should explore thoughts and feelings, as well as actions. The assessment interview should give some indication of the dangerousness of the abuser. Where denial is total and where physical violence has been used, the prognosis for rehabilitation is very poor. It is unlikely that children could be safe in the company of the abuser.

When there is some acceptance of responsibility, a programme of therapy, preferably both individual work and group work, may be helpful in enabling the abusers to control their illegal sexual actions. Treatment programmes in USA and Canada seem to show that the prognosis for offenders whose offences have been committed within a family setting, is better than for those who offend more indiscriminately. However, rehabilitation with a family should only be attempted if the abusers are able to demonstrate that there is an understanding of why they are a risk to children and have shown behavioural and emotional changes which reduce the risk of reoffending.

Child victim

Characteristics of abuse:

Relationship with abuser	Parent/carer Family friend/Relative Professional Stranger
Age of child	Chronological age Developmental status Physical or intellectual vulnerability
Quality of parenting	Good/good enough Neglectful Severe attachment problems
Type of abuse	Long term/regular Infrequent/single episode Violent/coerced Groomed/enticed Many abusers
Reaction of important others	Believing/supportive Unbelieving Rejecting
Other factors	Gender Ethnic origin Religion

Protection issues

Whether the child remains at home or is placed elsewhere will depend on whether the parents/carers believe the statement of abuse and are able to take protective action. Clearly the closer the child is to the abuser, the greater the likelihood that short term protection will have to be sought outside the child's home.

The age and vulnerability of the child will also play a part. It may be possible to leave an older child in a less protective environment if the child is clear that this is their preferred choice and shows self-protective ability. Similarly, good enough parenting will make it more possible to ensure the child stays at home. Even where the abuser is identified, the parents must be aware that their child may now be more vulnerable to other abusers and will still need help and protection. With insecurely attached children not only is the risk of reabuse greater but so is the emotional trauma of separation. These will have clear implications for protection and therapy. Children who have been enticed into long term abuse which has also met some of their emotional needs for nurture, will have very different protective issues from those who have had a short-term and violent abusive experience.

To ensure a protective environment for the child, it is essential to identify a number of basic components. These include identifying with the child an adult to whom they have easy access, whom they perceive as protective, and to whom they can turn if they feel threatened. Appropriate boundaries in family living should also be identified with the child. These would include rules about bathrooms and bedrooms — who enters with whom — as well as rules about clothes — is nudity around the house permissible?

Once the child understands at their developmental level these rules and also rules about touching and affection giving, and has identified their protective adult, they should be helped to work out a plan of action if they think the rules are broken.

Many of these topics can be discussed with the child as 'what if' questions:

'What if you meet Dad in the street?'
'What if you are bought secret presents?'
'What if Mum breaks the rules and Dad doesn't say anything?'
'What if you're touched in a way you don't like?'
'What if you're home on holiday and Uncle Billy comes around?'

Furthermore, and if possible, there should be discussion with the child about the signs they would give if they were abused again and felt they were unable to say. This could include discussion about their behaviour when they were being abused and had not been able to tell.

These issues and the ability of the child to cope, will usually be established over time. The age of the child and a supportive adult will be crucial to success and protection.

Therapy issues
Factors in the abuse which have been associated with trauma have been identified as age at onset of the abuse, length and frequency of abuse,

relationship with the abuser and number of abusers. While some researchers (see Wyatt and Powell 1988) suggest violence is associated with long term harm, Hindman (Hindman J 1989) indicates that a violent sexual assault is unlikely to result in distortion of the victim's perception of the event. The violence often enables the victim to identify the abusive element and may mean the victim is not enmeshed in a damaging scenario of self blame and taking responsibility. It would appear that the younger the victim and the longer the period of abuse, the more likely it is that the victim will adopt changes in behaviour and perception to accommodate the abuse. This will damage their own ability to develop normally.

General treatment issues identified both by Sgroi (1982) and MacFarlane et al (1986) include the 'damaged goods syndrome' often evident in the low self-esteem of victims, and guilt resultant, not only from participation in the sexual behaviour, but also from feeling responsible for the disruption consequent to disclosure. Fear is a third feature which may result in nightmares and clinging behaviour and stems from the verbal and physical threats of harm should they tell. Many victims exhibit an inability to trust adults, they may also be depressed and have poor social skills. However, others exhibit repressed anger and hostility with acting-out behaviour. They may also display role confusion and pseudomaturity. Many who have experienced long term abuse from an early age will have learnt to suppress their own emotions concentrating on pleasing adults.

Where the child has been abused by a non-family member and has good enough parents, the best therapist is often one of the child's parents guided and supported by a skilled professional. This may also be true of children placed in foster care, substituting the foster parent for a natural parent.

For older children individual work may be helpfully supplemented by group work. Indeed a combination of individual therapy and group work varied accordingly with the child's individual needs is usually the preferred mode of helping. Care should be taken to ensure that help is available over a period of time, not necessarily continuously, so that as new issues emerge at different stages of the child's progress to maturity, appropriate help is available in a flexible way.

Environmental factors

Characteristics of abuse:
Protective adult   Parent/mother

Reaction of professionals	Planned help
	Unplanned/incompetent
	Therapy programme
	Unsupportive/unbelieving
	Listening therapists
Reaction of community	Supportive/believing
	Unsupportive/rejecting
	Media publicity
	Sexual object
Legal process	Interviews
	Medical examination
	Court delays
	Court appearance

Protection issues

Contrary to popular myth, most mothers are not aware of on-going sexual abuse. Marriage demands considerable blind trust and denial for survival. A woman does not commit her life and security to a man she believes is capable of molesting his own children. The 'obvious' clues to sexual abuse are usually obvious only in retrospect. Our assumptions that the mother 'must have known' merely parallels the demand of the child that the mother must be in touch intuitively with invisible and even deliberately concealed family discomfort.

(Summit 1983)

Work with abusers has highlighted and underlined this judgement. Abusers may go to considerable lengths to ensure that the family environment is one in which abuse can flourish undetected.

The family could see no harm in him. He bails them out financially and provides things for the family. Clothes and a bike have been promised.

The stepparent who drives a wedge between natural parent and child ensuring the death of trust between them; the family friend who provides treats and extras; the school teacher who can target vulnerable children and point to home problems as the source of behaviour disturbance; all are able to hoodwink the child's environment and continue to abuse while diverting suspicion or labelling the child as a liar. It is not difficult to have a child labelled a liar. What chance then has the child that important others in the environment will believe the allegations of abuse?

And yet a believing, caring adult is the single most important factor in providing protection for the child. In any family there will be one, two or no non-abusing carers. Where there is one or more, the assessment of this parent will be crucial to decisions regarding the safest placement for a child. It will also influence the therapeutic programme arranged for the child and family.

The ideal would be a carer who believes the child's allegation, can sympathise with the child's dilemma, and help bring the situation to the attention of others who can enlist help. Such a carer will hold the perpetrator responsible for the abuse and cooperate with the statutory agencies to help to protect the child. This carer will not be dependent on the abuser for fulfilment of emotional needs but will be able to protect and nurture the child as a single parent supported by appropriate family and community networks.

At the other end of the scale, the worst situation will be a carer who disbelieves the child either denying the possibility of abuse or blaming the child as the seducer. This carer is unlikely to cooperate with the statutory agencies and may be highly dependent on the abuser for fulfilment of emotional and dependency needs. Additionally, the family will be isolated and without supportive networks either familial or community.

In reality, most carers will be somewhere on a continuum between the ideal and worst scenarios and may, with appropriate support, be moved into a more favourable position.

An acknowledgement of issues of loss and a non-judgemental approach will be essential to enable the non-abusing carer to accept and come to terms with the abuse and the abuser.

> 'She never judged us, and she was not negative towards my partner so I was able to talk about my hate and my love and my feelings of sorrow for him. She really understood all our confusion.' Carer of an abused child talking about their social worker.

While there must be an initial assessment, it should be remembered that people change. The non-abusing carer may move from a stance which believes the child and is supportive, to one which is unbelieving. Movement can also be in the other direction. The vital ingredient will be support and being allowed to express and sort out confusion. An attitude which blames, overtly or covertly, the non-abusing parent for being apparently unprotective is unlikely to be helpful to child or family. Such an attitude creates defensive hostility and may result in the carer regressing to a non-believing attitude.

As with abusers, therapy may be a combination of individual and group work. However, at least some experience of group therapy is likely to be very beneficial to the non-abusing parent. Perhaps this is also a field where self-help and voluntary support of others along the lines of *Parents United* (Giarretto 1982) could be explored further. In work with a group of parents whose adolescent sons were attending a parallel group for boys who had abused younger children, the parents moved from a position of minimisation and denial to some understanding of their sons' problems. All the members attended a recall group six months later and all expressed a willingness to be involved in supporting other parents in a similar position.

Unfortunately, in many areas there are not even ongoing group work facilities for victims of abuse, let alone their carers or other members of the family.

There is little doubt that a comprehensive programme which allows for group work, individual therapy, marital therapy, family therapy and work with siblings, is a rare, (and expensive) facility for only too many areas. However, some victims and families may not need this extensive programme. While the ultimate aim may be to provide comprehensive programmes, an ongoing group work programme for each group is probably the single most important element.

Other considerations

At some point, the child or their carer should be informed of the possibility of applying for criminal injuries compensation. There does not need to be a conviction, or even a named abuser. It is sufficient that abuse has occurred, is of sufficient gravity to qualify for compensation, the police have been informed, and an investigation undertaken. Advice regarding application can be obtained from the Police, Social Services, or the Citizens' Advice Bureau.

Should sexually abused children be specifically targeted for HIV/AIDS counselling? This strays into arguments about high risk groups which anger many health educationalists and pressure groups.

An attempt to counsel a group of abused boys as part of a post-abuse recovery group proved unhelpful in that they were unable to ask specific questions in front of the group. Since sexual abuse victims already carry the stigma of abuse and many suffer jibes from peers, to further stigmatise by picking them out as a target group for counselling seems unwise. Education about the risk of AIDS as well as other sexually transmitted diseases should be available as part of all school health education programmes. In addition, there should be a clear and confidential route for counselling at the request of the child.

Presently there are no indications that the rate of HIV/AIDS infection in victims of abuse is significant (Fost 1990). Inevitably, as the infection spreads in society this group, as with any group experiencing unprotected sex, will be vulnerable. It has yet to be recorded that the abuser wore a condom to protect the child from infection.

experiencing unprotected sex, will be vulnerable. It has yet to be recorded that the abuser wore a condom to protect the child from infection.

Summary

- Issues of a comprehensive assessment.

- Issues of protection and treatment; and

- Place for HIV/AIDS education counselling is briefly discussed.

References and bibliography

Fost, 1990 Ethical considerations in testing victims of sexual abuse for HIV infection. *Child abuse and neglect* **14**: 5–7.

Giarretto, 1982 *Integrated treatment of child sexual abuse: a treatment and training manual.* Science and Behaviour Books, Palo Alto, CA.

Hindman J, 1989 *Just before dawn: trauma assessment and sexual victimisation.* Alexandria Associates, US.

Luborsky L et al, 1986 Do therapists vary much in their success? Findings of four outcome studies. *American Orthopsychiatric Association* pp501–12.

MacFarlane K, Waterman J et al, 1986 *Sexual abuse of young children.* Guilford Press, US.

Sgroi S, Blick L and Porter F, 1982 A conceptual framework for child sexual abuse. In Sgroi S (ed) *Handbook of clinical intervention in child sexual abuse.* Lexington Books.

Summit, R C, 1983 The child sexual abuse accommodation syndrome. *Child abuse and neglect* **7**: 177–93.

Wills D, 1983 Approaching the incestuous and sexually abusive family. *Journal of Adolescence* **6**: 229–46.

Wyatt G E and Powell G J (ed) 1988 *Lasting effects of child sexual abuse.* Sage Focus Publications, US.

8 Legal context

Criminal context

While most acts which constitute sexual abuse will also be against the law, only a small percentage of known cases will result in prosecution. It is generally acknowledged that the real extent of sex offending, whether it be against children or adults, is greatly in excess of the number who are brought to justice.

According to the crime statistics for 1989 in England and Wales, 3,898 men and 23 women were sentenced by magistrates courts for indictable sexual offences. A further 3,280 men and 52 women were sentenced at Crown Court. One thousand and forty-eight men were also sentenced for indecent exposure. These statistics do not distinguish between offences against adults and offences against children, only by type of offence. For example, 1,193 were dealt with in magistrates courts for indecency between males.

The total prison population in 1989 was 36,734 of whom 2,982 had been convicted of sex offences (HM Inspectorate of Probation).

A brief outline of sexual offences relating most commonly to children, together with maximum length of sentence may helpfully put these figures into context.

Legal context

Unlawful sexual intercourse
A man may not have intercourse with a girl under the age of sixteen, whether or not she consents. Penetration to any degree constitutes an offence. It is a defence in respect of girls aged 14 to 16 years if:

1. The man is aged under 24, has not been charged with a similar offence and reasonably believes the girl was aged sixteen or over.

2. The couple were married in a country which permits marriage below
    the age of 16 even though the marriage is invalid in this country.
                                                (Sexual Offences Act 1956.)

Rape
This is forcible sexual intercourse and consent by a child is immaterial.
The intercourse need not be complete in that penetration of any
degree is enough to prove rape. (*Sexual Offences Act* 1956 amended
1976.)

Incest
Again consent is immaterial in that incest is defined by the relationship
between the partners. Both partners are deemed in law to be equally
guilty. The defined relationships are:

1. A man to have intercourse with a woman he knows to be his daughter,
    granddaughter, sister, half-sister or mother.

2. A woman aged 16 or over to have intercourse with a man she knows to
    be her father, grandfather, brother, half-brother or son.
                                                (*Sexual Offences Act* 1956.)

It is also an offence for a man to incite a girl under sixteen to have an
incestuous sexual relationship. (*Criminal Law Act* 1977.)

Buggery
This covers partial or complete penetration of the anus and is illegal
apart from consenting males in private who are aged 21 or over. (*Sexual
Offences Act* 1956 as amended 1967.)

Assault with intent to commit buggery
In many cases where buggery cannot be proved, this charge will be
used. (*Sexual Offences Act* 1956.)

Gross indecency
While physical contact is not always necessary, this term refers only to
acts of indecency between males. It is, however, more likely to cover
such actions as mutual masturbation, oral-genital contact, etc but may
include, for example, procuring for the commission of the act. (*Sexual
Offences Act* 1956 amended 1967.)

Indecent assault
The emphasis here is on the word assault which implies use of force and

lack of consent, combined with physical contact in circumstances of indecency. This could, for example, include touching a child while suggesting a sexual act. (*Sexual Offences Act* 1956.)

Indecent conduct with or towards a child
This covers those offences when the person either commits an indecent act with a child under 14 years, or incites the child to commit such an act. This could cover such offences as asking the child to masturbate the adult, or inducing the child to perform sexual acts with another child. (*Indecency with Children Act* 1960.)

There are also provisions covering the taking of indecent photographs of children (*Protection of Children Act* 1978) and causing or encouraging prostitution with a girl of 16 or under. (*Sexual Offences Act* 1956.)

There are certain inconsistencies, for example, illegitimate children are covered by the laws on incest, but adopted or step children are not. Father/son relationships are covered by the offences of buggery and indecent assault but not those of incest. However, by applying the correct act it is theoretically possible to prosecute most acts of sexual abuse.

There are also inconsistencies concerning age and gender with regard to whether a sexual act will be regarded as illegal, as opposed to abusive. Thus a 16 year old girl is deemed able to consent to sexual intercourse. A 16 year old boy is not able to consent to a sexual relationship with another male and must wait until both partners are aged 21, or risk placing his older partner in jeopardy with the law.

When it comes to prosecution however, the primary problem lies in the area of proving the abuse beyond reasonable doubt. Normally the only witnesses will be the abuser and the victim, and there is but rarely collaborative evidence. For a discussion of the difficulties of prosecution and law relating to child witnesses *see* Spencer J R and Flin R (1990).

Sentences
Despite the difficulties of prosecution and the law, penalties can be severe (BASPCAN 1981):

Offence:	**Maximum sentence:**
Rape	Life
Buggery	Life
Unlawful sexual intercourse:	
with a girl under 13	Life
with a girl under 16	2 years

Indecent assault against:
a male	10 years
a girl under 13 years	5 years
a girl under 16 years	2 years

Indecency with or towards a child under 14 years	2 years
Incest	2 years to life according to gender and age

Criminal Justice Act 1991
(See also Home Office Circular 88/91)

The provisions of this Act, which will mainly come into operation during October 1992, will have an effect both on sentencing and evidence in child sexual abuse cases. The Act recognises the distinction between crimes against property and those against persons. It suggests that custodial sentences may be more appropriate for the latter in order to protect the public from serious harm.

In future, discretionary parole will be replaced by automatic release on licence, (except where remission is lost) at the halfway point of the sentence, for sentences up to four years. This release will be discretionary for prisoners serving longer than four years. However, when the conviction has been for a sexual offence, and the conviction has been for 12 months or more, the sentencing court may require the offender to be supervised on licence from the point of release until the end of the sentence. This should enable better and longer supervision of sex offenders resulting in greater protection for children. An offender on licence may be recalled to prison for breach of licence conditions.

There are also significant changes in the rules regulating children's evidence.

The new rules cover situations where the child is a victim or witness in situations where either a sexual or violent crime is alleged.

Until the implementation of the Act, children have been judged not to be competent witnesses. Before they were able to give evidence they were required to be specially examined by the judge with particular reference to their knowledge and understanding of telling the truth. This will no longer be required and the jury will decide what weight they wish to place on the child's evidence.

This may lead to a helpful change in attitudes and the realisation that children can be competent witnesses. Of still greater significance are the moves designed to lessen the trauma of a court appearance for the child.

A videotape of the investigative interview may be used in evidence instead of requiring the child to repeat this evidence orally. The child may still be required to come to court to be cross-examined but such cross-examinations will take place with the child outside the court room via a TV link. This will ensure that the child is not confronted with the alleged abuser in a face-to-face court room situation. In the past, some such confrontations have so terrified or upset the child that the trial has had to be stopped and the case dismissed. These provisions place a great responsibility on police and social workers to ensure that all investigative interviews are videotaped and conducted in a way which conforms to the rules of evidence. Guidance for conducting these interviews is to be issued — possibly in August 1992 — by the Home Office in conjunction with the Department of Health.

Helpfully the Act imposes a clear duty on the courts to ensure that there is no unnecessary delay in getting the cases to court. If this can be done, not only might the child's evidence be clearer but it may be possible to undertake all aspects of therapeutic work with the child at an earlier stage without risking allegations of contamination of the child's evidence.

Decision to prosecute

The evidential requirement for criminal proceedings is proof beyond reasonable doubt. The burden of proof lies with the prosecution. Unless there is a confession, evidence needs to be corroborated. Frequently, in cases of child sexual abuse the only evidence available is that of the child's statement which cannot be corroborated in any other way. Consequently, only a small proportion of cases actually come to court.

The decision to initiate criminal proceedings rests with the Crown Prosecution Service. The decision will be based on whether there is sufficient substantial evidence to prosecute; whether it is in the public interest that there should be proceedings against a particular alleged offender; and whether it is in the best interests of the child victim that proceedings be taken. In making their decision, the Crown Prosecution Service will listen to the recommendations of the police. In many areas, the police recommendations will incorporate the views of those working with the child, and/or the recommendations of a Child Protection Conference.

The standard of proof in civil courts is one of balance of probabilities. The court will make an order which focuses on promoting the best interest of the child. For all these reasons, where legal measures are necessary to protect children, the more likely route will be via civil courts and the *Children Act* 1989 rather than through criminal proceedings and the prosecution of the offenders.

Children Act 1989

The implementation of the *Children Act* in October 1991 brought a fundamental change in approach to many aspects of the law relating to children. For the purposes of working with children alleged to have been abused, it is important to understand those sections of the Act which relate to the powers and duties of local authorities, the ways in which children can be protected, and the areas relating to consent to medical treatment. Throughout the Act there are the fundamental assumptions: that parents are responsible for their children; that local authorities will work in partnership with parents to enable them to exercise their parental responsibility in the best interest of the child; and that children are best brought up within their own families so long as it is safe to do so. The emphasis of the Act is on working in partnership with parents on a voluntary basis.

Underlying principles
These are that a Court will only make an order if this appears to be better for the child than making no order. In all cases when the Court determines any question with respect to the child's upbringing, the child's welfare must be the paramount consideration.

This means that before making an order the Court must consider a number of factors constituting a *Welfare Checklist*. These are:

1. The ascertainable wishes and feelings of the child.

2. The child's physical, emotional and educational needs.

3. The likely effects on the child of any changes in the child's circumstances.

4. The child's age, gender, race and background and any other characteristics the Court may feel relevant.

5. Any harm the child has suffered or is at risk of suffering.

6. How capable each of the child's parents is of meeting the child's needs.

7. The range of powers available to the court in the proceedings in question.

(Children Act 1989)

This Welfare Checklist has been devised for the courts in deciding the future of children. It is entirely appropriate for social workers and others such as counsellors to keep it to the forefront of their minds when making decisions such as advice regarding HIV/AIDS counselling and testing.

Parental responsibility

I the past it may have seemed conveniently easy to ignore absent parents when making decisions about children, particularly when they had had no contact over a period of time. However, it is now necessary to understand the concept of parental responsibility and ensure that all the appropriate carers have been consulted if it is possible to do so, with regard, for example, to permission for medical treatment.

Once a person has parental responsibility acquired by means of an order, they will only lose that responsibility if the order is discharged or expires. Birth mothers and fathers married to the birth mother at or after the time of conception automatically have parental responsibility and only lose it if the child is adopted. An unmarried father may acquire parental responsibility by going to court for an order or by voluntary arrangement with the birth mother. Others may acquire it through a court order, although one person acquiring responsibility does not remove another's responsibility. The making of a Care Order gives Social Services Departments parental responsibility. This responsibility they must share with the parents. The parent's responsibility may only be limited if it is necessary to safeguard or promote the child's welfare.

The phrase 'parental responsibility' replaces the concept of 'parental rights' and is defined in the Act as 'the rights, duties, powers, responsibilities and authority which a parent has in relation to the child and the childs property'.

The implications of this for professional practice are that before a referral for HIV/AIDS counselling or testing is made, or accepted, the following questions should be asked:

1. Who has parental responsibility?

2. Is the child subject to a court order?

3. What are the directions of the court, if any, in relation to this referral?

4. Who has the right to consent to the referral?

5. What are the views of the child?

Powers and duties of the local authority

The local authority has a general duty to safeguard and promote the welfare of children, within their area, who are in need.

The local authority also has the specific duty to investigate when there is reasonable cause to suspect that a child is suffering, or is likely to suffer, significant harm.

This investigation should include an objective assessment of the needs of the child, including the risk of abuse, the need for protection, and the family's ability to meet these needs.

The Act lays a duty on the other professionals to assist the local authority in their enquiries by providing relevant information and advice if called upon to do so. However, the other professionals are not required to comply with this request if, given all the circumstances of the case, it appears unreasonable to do so. The other professionals specified by the Act are employees of any local authority, any local education authority and any health authority or NHS trust.

This has implications with regard to confidentiality which are discussed later in this chapter.

In the course of the investigation the local authority will either try to ensure that the child is seen by a social worker, or by another person, possibly from an agency already visiting the family, who is authorised by the local authority for this purpose.

Where the local authority is unable to obtain access to the child, they must apply for a court order unless they are satisfied that the child's welfare can be safeguarded without such an order.

Court orders

In emergency situations when the court is satisfied that the child is likely to suffer significant harm, an *Emergency Protection Order* (E.P.O.) will be granted, either to remove the child from the presence of danger, or to prevent the child being moved to a potentially dangerous situation.

This order is initially only for eight days and may be discharged by application after 72 hours. The court may also make directions regarding contact with the child and/or medical or psychiatric examination or assessment.

In non-emergency situations where there is concern that a child may be suffering, or is likely to suffer, significant harm and where the child's parents are unwilling voluntarily to cooperate with an assessment of the child's situation, the local authority can apply for a *Child Assessment Order.*

It is unlikely that an application for this order will be made without interagency agreement. The court will make decisions regarding outline plans for medical, psychological and social assessment which must be completed within seven days from the commencement of the order. While the child's carers will be expected to cooperate, in so far as they must produce the child for assessment and provide a social/medical history of the child, the child may refuse to cooperate with the assessment process. The guidance document covering this section of the Act specifically points out that all professionals should avoid coercing the child into agreement to cooperate even where there is a belief that the refusal to cooperate is a product of coercion by a carer or friend. (*Children Act* 1989 Guidance and Regulations Vol. 1.)

It is unlikely that referral for HIV/AIDS counselling will form part of such an initial assessment. The principle of the child's right to refuse to cooperate is an important one which must be borne in mind when giving consideration to a referral for counselling. The child's desires and wishes in the process must be carefully checked.

There will be situations where it is considered not to be in the child's best interests for the child to remain or return home to the immediate family. In this situation a *Care Order* will be sought by the local authority. A Care Order should be sought only when there appears to be no better way of safeguarding and promoting the welfare of the child suffering, or likely to suffer, significant harm.

The grounds for the order are:

(i)   That the child concerned is suffering or is likely to suffer significant harm; and

(ii) That the harm or likelihood of harm is attributable to:
    (a) the care given to the child or likely to be given to the child, if the order were not made, not being what would be reasonable to expect a parent to give to the child, or
    (b) the child is beyond parental control.

(Children Act 1989)

Once the order is granted, the local authority acquires parental responsibility which is shared by the parents, but the local authority has the power to decide the extent to which the parents may exercise their parental responsibility to the child.

The child in care may be looked after by the local authority and placed in, for example, a foster home. On the other hand, a child may be placed in a local authority foster home at the request of the child's parents who will retain full parental responsibility for the child. Here again it will be necessary for the counsellor to be clear who has parental responsibility and who, besides the child, should be consulted about HIV/AIDS counselling.

The situation may be further complicated by the fact that a child subject to a court order will also have a court appointed guardian ad litem whose role is to safeguard the child's wishes and best interests. It may be wise to consult the child's guardian also if this is the situation, particularly with younger children not deemed able to make informed decisions for themselves.

Medical examination: consent to treatment

It has been increasingly recognised that children both want and need to make decisions for themselves, and that the exercise of choice is essential for the development of the child's sense of responsibility. This means that carers have to face the fact that children must make choices but may sometimes make wrong choices which inevitably have painful consequences. This is particularly difficult where the child has been abused and is vulnerable to further hurt. Allowing such children the freedom to make choices even if they are wrong becomes the more difficult for caring adults.

In practice, allowing children to make choices involves: giving them more and better information; allowing them to consult with different people; and being clear as to which choices are appropriate for children at what age and which are not.

Children of 16 and over are able to give their own consent to medical treatment, although it is now less clear whether they are able to refuse medical treatment against their parent's wishes in certain circumstances (*R&R 19913WLR592*).

Children under 16 may also be able to give or refuse consent depending on whether they are able to understand the full implications of the nature of the treatment. However, 'R&R' makes the situation of the child of less than 16 who withholds consent for medical treatment somewhat problematic. There appears to be a conflict between this judgement and the philosophy of the *Children Act*. In cases of doubt, all practitioners will need to obtain clear legal advice. In practice, when it comes to medical examination for children who are suspected to have been sexually abused, it is unlikely that any doctor familiar with abuse and its effects will press examination on even a young child for other than clear medical necessity.

It is perhaps helpful to see the child's participation in decision making as part of a continuum ranging from a decision within the capacity of the child, if they are given appropriate information; through a joint decision making process, where the adult consults with the child; to those situations where the adult makes the decision and the child is informed. At no point on this continuum should the child be given unrealistic expectations about their role in making decisions. Conversely, at no time should they be excluded from information which, when properly presented at the appropriate developmental level, would allow them to make informed choices, or understand why the adult has made the choice. This is particularly important with abused children who will have had no choice as to whether they participated in the sexual activity, but who will frequently have been presented with a pseudochoice situation which has implied that they were both responsible and made the choice to participate. In the abusive situation they will not have been presented with either full information or alternatives. In subsequent situations they will need to be able to discuss alternatives and understand the consequences of choices between the alternatives.

Within this scenario, special provision will need to be made for children with communication difficulties. These children will include not only those for whom English may be a second language, but also those children with sensory or educational handicaps which impair their ability to communicate. In all these situations it may be necessary to look at special arrangements to facilitate communication.

It may be that guidelines for referring children under the age of 16 for HIV/AIDS counselling or testing should be little different from the general guidelines which are given to general practitioners faced with a request to provide under 16 year olds with contraceptive advice and treatment.

In outline these suggest that special care should be taken not to undermine parental responsibility and there should be a discussion with the young person about the advisability of talking to their parent/carer of their wish for HIV testing.

If this approach fails, it is suggested that referral for counselling should be made if it is considered that the young person not only understands the advice, but has the maturity to understand the implications, and it is in their best interests to receive counselling about HIV testing.

In any event, any court orders in relation to the child must be borne in mind when coming to a decision.

Confidentiality and record keeping

The emphasis of this book has primarily centred on the victim of abuse. However, the situation may arise for social workers and counsellors to work with adults with HIV/AIDS where they believe that the adult is engaged in a relationship with a child, or is addicted to paedophilic activity. In these circumstances, what is their responsibility to the children who may be at risk? There is not, and probably never will be, an easy answer. Practitioners should beware of slipping into secretive, collusive, relationships with clients which may undermine their duty to their agency. This is especially so when they belong to a statutory agency charged with responsibility for protecting children.

It should always be made clear that if the counsellor or social worker, is employed by the local authority or health authority, their duty to protect children overrides their normal rules of confidentiality. There can frequently be a confusion between confidentiality and secrecy.

The worker in this situation does not operate independently but as a member of a team and in an agency with a line manager. In these circumstances, such information is appropriately shared with the line manager. The client should be aware from the outset that some information will be shared on a 'need to know' basis.

In one situation of this kind, the information that a Schedule 1 offender, who had a long history of sexual offences against children, was probably HIV positive, was relayed anonymously to a Social Services Department. Initially contact was made through the hospital social work department to the consultant treating the offender. A request was made that the consultant should discuss the implications of the illness and implications for past victims with the offender. Had this approach not been successful, a social worker would, of necessity, have discussed the information with the offender. In this instance two services were able to use their separate information bases to clarify the situation. Frequently the professionals dealing with HIV/AIDS related issues will be unaware that there may also be issues relating to the protection of children. They must keep an open mind to the possibility.

In this instance the situation was brought to notice by the anonymous referral. Several approaches to resolving the conflict between protecting children and preserving confidentiality are possible and need to be examined prior to the situation arising. A simple solution is to do nothing. This approach is unacceptable because it will probably leave children unprotected.

Alternatively, the practitioner can ignore the possible conflict hoping the situation will never arise. Such a solution will lead to *ad hoc* solutions which may also run the risk of being unsuccessful either at protecting the children or preserving confidentiality.

Perhaps the most successful approach is interagency liaison to agree guidelines regarding confidentiality before the problem arises. These could, for example, provide complete confidentiality for the victim to discuss their abuse with the counsellor regardless of any statements to police or social worker. This may also include an agreement that no records would be kept.

On the other hand, for alleged offenders, the procedures could allow for guidance and persuasion, with agreement for non-prosecution for past offences hitherto undisclosed, to ensure that there is full knowledge of victims and their abuse. With such knowledge the victims can be given help appropriate to their needs.

In both situations, health, social services and police need to have procedures which put the best interests of the child victim before all other considerations.

Summary

- This chapter looks briefly at sexual offences as defined within the legal system indicating maximum sentences and some inconsistencies.

- The legal situation with regard to protection of children is outlined looking at the Welfare Checklist, parental responsibility and relevant orders obtainable within the current legislative framework of the *Children Act* 1989.

- The child's right to make decisions and issues of confidentiality are discussed in detail in Section 3 from the social work viewpoint of the protection of children and the therapeutic value of self-determination for young people

- The dilemma of treating abusers who have HIV/AIDS is discussed with suggestions for alternative solutions.

References and bibliography

BASPCAN (1981). Child Sexual Abuse

Children Act 1989— In particular Guidance and Regulations Volume 1 — Court Orders.

Criminal Justice Act 1991 General Guide Home Office Circular 88/91.

Criminal Law Act 1977.

HM Inspectorate of Probation *The Work of the Probation Service With Sex Offenders. Report of a Thematic Inspection.* (July 1991). HMSO.

Indecency with Children Act 1960.

Protection of Children Act 1978.

R&R 19913WLR592.

Sexual Offences Act 1956.

Sexual Offences Act 1956 amended 1976.

Spencer, J R and Flin R, 1990 *The evidence of children. The law and psychology.* Blackstone Press Ltd.

Section 3 AIDS AND COUNSELLING

Introduction

The first two chapters of this section aim to give the practitioner the necessary background information about the human immuno-deficiency virus (HIV) and its relationship to the acquired immune deficiency syndrome (AIDS). Treatment issues are not covered as they are changing rapidly in the light of new drug trials and are best left to those professionals dealing with the medical care of the child. The resources section following chapter 14 mentions a manual with a particularly good medical reference guide for those professionals requiring specialist knowledge.

Chapters 11 and 12 deal with the sociological and legal issues appertaining to HIV and are intended to guide and assist the practitioner to make informed choices for practice.

Chapter 13 addresses the need for guidelines to be in place prior to offering a counselling service. Chapter 14 examines the counselling session and discusses possible outcomes for the child and practitioner.

A reference section has been included at the end of this section suggesting useful books, workpacks and organisations which may be of assistance in the learning process of practitioner or child.

9 AIDS and related issues

Anyone involved in AIDS counselling with a child who has been sexually abused will need to have some understanding of HIV/AIDS but will not necessarily need the huge amount of specialist knowledge required by a consultant with special responsibility for treatment of HIV/AIDS.

Good communication skills and empathy, together with a broad basic understanding of HIV and its implications, are far more important than impressive qualifications.

This chapter aims to look at the basic facts about HIV, and to explain the difference between AIDS and HIV, in order to help the practitioner begin to help the child.

What is HIV?

HIV stands for Human Immunodeficiency Virus. It is now generally accepted that it is probably this virus which causes the immune system of an individual to become severely compromised, and which may result in the syndrome commonly known as AIDS.

Put quite simply, the virus may attack and destroy the immune system leaving it vulnerable to infections and diseases that would not normally have an opportunity to develop.

What is AIDS?

AIDS stands for Acquired Immune Deficiency Syndrome.

Acquired	generally not present at birth
Immune Deficiency	impairment of the body's defence system
Syndrome	collection of specific conditions and infections

It is diagnosed by the patient fulfilling a set of clinical criteria which include opportunistic or life threatening infections.

Again, put quite simply, AIDS is the worst possible consequence of infection by HIV, but it is not the only consequence. At present there are a range of possible scenarios which may occur as a result of infection by HIV:

Acute HIV infection
Asymptomatic HIV infection
Persistent generalised lymphadenopathy
Symptomatic HIV infection
Acquired immune deficiency syndrome

When a person becomes infected with HIV, they may experience a slight fever, headache or rash, and feel generally unwell for a brief period. This is known as *Acute HIV Infection* and may last perhaps one to four weeks.

Many people experience no symptoms at all after contracting the virus, but are still infectious. This is known as *Asymptomatic HIV infection* and can last for some years.

Persistent generalised lymphadenopathy (PGL) is a common occurrence. This is identified by the presence of enlarged lymph nodes in two or more places on the body, excluding the groin area. Since many people have enlarged lymph nodes at some time during their life, it should not be assumed that this alone means that they have HIV infection.

Early education about HIV and AIDS included the term AIDS related complex (ARC). In terms of AIDS education, perhaps a more useful term of reference for ARC is *HIV related illness, or Symptomatic HIV infection.*

Some, or any of these, may indicate symptomatic HIV infection:

Fever
Night sweats that are heavy or prolonged
Unexplained weight loss
Chronic fatigue
Diarrhoea
Oral Thrush
Herpes
Bleeding gums

All of the above can be successfully treated by medication and can occur in people who are not infected with HIV. However, in a person who is HIV positive, they are generally much more severe.

Likewise, early educationalists also talked about 'full-blown' AIDS.

This tended to imply that there may be a 'half-blown' version. AIDS differs from HIV related illness in that life threatening infections and tumours are now taking the opportunity to attack a *severely* damaged immune system, but the term 'full-blown' AIDS is misleading and should be avoided.

The three most commonly seen opportunistic, or life threatening infections in AIDS, tend to be:

pneumonia known as *Pneumocystis carinii Pneumonia* (PCP);
skin cancer known as Kaposi's Sarcoma (KS); and
virus related to herpes called Cytomegalovirus (CMV).

These are by no means the only opportunistic infections and TB or brain tumours are just two of many more diseases which may occur when the immune system is failing.

Pneumocystis carinii pneumonia, prior to the days of AIDS, tended to be seen only in people with weak immune systems due to drug therapy or who had other severe diseases. These days it is commonly seen in people with AIDS and if treatment is given at an early stage, there is a good chance of recovery. At the time of writing, the mortality rate for PCP is now as low as five per cent.

Kaposi's Sarcoma, prior to AIDS, accounted for less than one per cent of all cancers (Daniels 1986). It is now the most common tumour in people with AIDS and appears as purply pink skin lesions or blotches which are slightly raised and generally painless. They can occur anywhere on the body and occur independently of each other. Psychologically, KS can be damaging as it is a constant reminder of AIDS. If it occurs internally (lungs, lymph nodes, intestine) this is physically more serious (Conlon 1988).

Cytomegalovirus can occur in anyone with a damaged immune system, e.g. after organ transpants. In people with AIDS it can present in three ways by infecting:

1. eyes causing cytomegalovirus retinitis and blindness
2. intestines and gullet
3. lungs

HIV may also act directly on the *central nervous system* by entering the brain across the blood brain barrier. This may happen independently of AIDS (Burton 1988) and symptoms may vary from a mild encephalitis or fever, to rapid progressive dementia. There may also be motor dysfunction creating difficulty in walking and talking, with perhaps some behavioural changes. The virus has also been known to affect the *heart muscle* directly, again independently of AIDS; causing heart disease which may result in death (*Lancet* 1991).

Progression of HIV infection

Young children and old people may have a more rapid progression to symptomatic HIV illness than others because of weak immune systems. However, in the main, most do not become ill for at least three years, and some who have been infected for longer than eight years are still free of illness (Terrence Higgins Trust 1991).

Evidence from the Communicable Disease Surveillance Centre, June 1989, would indicate that 50 per cent of those who are HIV infected will progress to AIDS within 10 years, and that without treatment, a further 20–30 per cent will have some HIV related conditions (Terrence Higgins Trust 1991).

These figures may change as new evidence becomes available as a result of research and time. It has only been 11 years since AIDS was first diagnosed, and only in 1983 was HIV identified as the virus involved. Those wishing to read more about the medical and scientific issues may find the Resources section of this book a useful guide.

Whilst not pretending that being diagnosed as having HIV infection is good news, neither should it be seen as an automatic death sentence. At present, many people are living with the virus and living lives of quality. Unfortunate media coverage may frequently do more psychological damage to a person with HIV than will the effects of the virus. Perhaps some inaccurate media coverage can be blamed on a lack of subject knowledge, however, that is possibly being too charitable and maybe most sensationalist stories are simply to sell papers. The person in the street may feel apprehensive and frightened by these stories, yet may also feel well informed. It is often difficult to ask a person to reexamine received wisdom and to become open to the realities of HIV as opposed to the popular mythology of the day.

Younger children may also have some confusion about HIV but are generally more able to acknowledge and accept new ideas and information. Their parents and guardians may need more time to work through the maze. This is not something which can be rushed and the practitioner will need to be firm about planning time for educative/ counselling sessions. The practitioner should remember that they are there for the client and must resist pressure from anyone to 'get it over with and then we can get on'. If it is important to address HIV as an issue, then it is important to do it properly.

In what is the virus transmitted?

Although the virus can be isolated in many fluids which are present in the body, there are very few in which it is transmitted.

At present it is known that HIV can be transmitted in:

Blood
Semen
Vaginal fluid
Breast milk

HIV has not been transmitted by contact with:

Saliva
Urine
Faeces
Vomit
Tears
Sweat
Skin (with the exception of skin grafts).

It may also be transmitted in blood products unless these have been heat treated. This is more of a common occurrence abroad. In the past, in Britain, those with haemophilia who were given Factor VIII, a blood clotting agent, were at risk of HIV infection. Approximately one fifth of these with haemophilia in Britain contracted HIV this way. These days all Factor VIII is heat treated and this should no longer happen.

Most common routes of transmission for HIV are:

Unprotected vaginal/anal intercourse
Sharing needles which puncture the skin
Mother to baby via the placenta
Infected blood or blood products

Virus is not transmitted by:

Sharing cups, glasses, cutlery
Swimming pools
Toilet seats
Kissing
Shaking hands
Hugging
Receiving the communion chalice
Donating blood (in the UK)
Coughing or sneezing
Headlice, mosquitos, fleas
Normal social contact in day to day living.

IIn order for there to be any risk of contracting HIV at all, it is necessary to have three things present:

1. the virus;
2. a fluid in which the virus is known to be transmitted; and
3. a point of entry into the bloodstream.

It is also necessary that the virus is alive. Virus which is exposed to the open air will rapidly break down and become nonviable after prolonged exposure. If HIV is assumed to be always present, it can be seen that both of the other criteria need to be met in order to be judged a risk situation for HIV infection as shown in Figure 3.9.1.

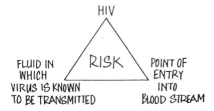

Figure 3.9.1   Triangle of risk

If only two of the criteria are met, then it can be assumed that there is little likelihood of possible HIV infection as in Figure 3.9.2.

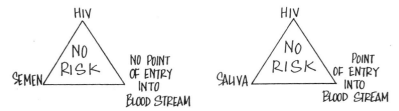

Figure 3.9.2   Triangles of risk — two criteria met

The 'triangle of risk' is a useful way of checking out many perceived HIV risk situations.

Risk group or risk activity?

In the early days of AIDS education, there were those who felt that it was sensible to talk about the risk *groups* in terms of HIV transmission, i.e. gay men/injecting drug users.

This was, in retrospect, ill-considered advice, as it is not who we are, or what label society tags us with that is the issue here. The issue is what we do as individuals in terms of risk *activity.*

Thus, anyone who takes part in unprotected vaginal or anal intercourse may be at risk of contracting HIV infection, no matter how that person's sexuality is defined.

Likewise, any person who allows their skin to be punctured by needles which have been used by or on others, may also be at risk of contracting the virus. This may include:

Injecting drugs
acupuncture
earpiercing
tatooing
electrolysis
medically related treatment in some countries

Many injectors of illicit drugs take advantage of needle exchange schemes which are usually available in larger towns and cities. These schemes should not be viewed as encouraging people to inject drugs, but rather as a positive attempt to stop the spread of HIV infection.

Most recognised practitioners of acupuncture, electrolysis, earpiercing and tattooing adhere very strictly to control of infection guidelines. However, it does no harm to check on this if attending as a client and go elsewhere if unhappy with a less than helpful response.

Children need to understand that to practise ear-piercing or tattooing on each other is a risky business and may result at best in a localised infection, and at worst HIV or Hepatitis B infection. The practice of becoming blood brothers or sisters by cutting skin and mingling blood, is also to be discouraged and may provide an opportunity for some useful educative work.

However, for the child who has been sexually abused, the main concern will be the nature of the abuse and whether or not it could be seen as an HIV risk.

The only effective way of preventing HIV transmission during penetrative intercourse is by wearing a condom. This reduces transmission by over 90 per cent if the condom has been treated with *Nonoxynol 9*®, a very effective spermicide, and if the condom is put on carefully (*see* chapter 11). It is rare for men who have intercourse with children to use condoms, and in the main the issue is one of unprotected, penetrative, sexual intercourse, the most common way of passing on HIV throughout the world today.

References

Burton, 1988 HIV and the Central Nervous System. *PSYNAPSE*, Newsletter of Neuropsychological Interest Group Issue 6.

Conlon, 1988 AIDS and HIV Infection. *British Medical Bulletin* **44** (1): 107 Churchill Livingstone.

Daniels Dr V G, 1986 *AIDS Q&A*. Cambridge Medical Books p42.

Lancet, 1991 **337** (May 18): 1215–16

Terrence Higgins Trust, 1991 *HIV & AIDS medical briefing*. p20.

10 HIV antibody testing

What are antibodies?

Antibodies are proteins produced in the blood in response to toxins or viral infection, in an attempt to fight off infection and neutralise the virus. They are merely 'markers' or 'footprints in the snow' that show that the infection has passed that way. Hence testing for the presence of antibodies is a way of checking whether a person may have been infected with HIV.

The process of the body producing antibodies to HIV is known as *seroconversion:*

1. Most people who become infected with HIV produce antibodies within 12 weeks of infection;

   However...

2. A few people may take up to two years to produce antibodies;

3. Some people never produce antibodies at all;

4. Some people lose antibodies to HIV but remain infected with the virus.

Antibodies to HIV infection appear to be ineffective, and so far, have not been able to neutralise the virus. So it can be seen that whether a person falls into the first, second, third or fourth group they would still, if infected, be able to pass that virus on to others.

Antibody testing

When a person has an HIV antibody test, a small amount of blood is taken, from the arm or other suitable site. This blood is then tested for antibodies to the virus. It is not an *AIDS Test* and to think of it as such will only cause confusion. It is simply a test which will detect the presence of antibodies which may have been produced by the body in an attempt to fight off HIV infection. It does not detect the presence of the virus itself. If antibodies are seen to be present, the person tested will be known as *HIV antibody positive or HIV+*. If no antibodies are detected, the person will be known as *HIV antibody negative or HIV−*.

If the result of the antibody test is positive, it should be assumed that the individual has the virus, is able to infect other people with it under certain circumstances (see chapter 9), and may already have done so. A positive result does not mean that a doctor can predict if, or when, an individual may develop symptoms of HIV infection. Some people remain well for a period of years after becoming HIV+, some produce minor illnesses, and others may develop AIDS.

If the result of the test is negative then antibodies to HIV have not been detected. This means one of two things:

1. The person has never been infected with HIV; or

2. The person may have been infected, but it is too early for antibodies to be detected.

As mentioned earlier, antibodies may take about 12 weeks to develop from the time of infection. This period is known as the *window period* when a person has not yet developed antibodies, but nevertheless remains infected and able to transmit the virus to others. If, after a second test, a negative result is given then it is *probable* that HIV infection has not occurred.

However, because some individuals take longer to produce antibodies than others, and some never produce any at all, it would be sensible to continue with safer sexual (or other) practice. False negatives do occur, and a person may be infectious to others even in the absence of antibodies.

Who will take blood for testing?

Taking blood for testing for HIV antibodies can take place at a GP surgery or at a Genitourinary (GU) or sexually transmitted diseases (STD) clinic. The results of the test usually take anything from one day to three weeks depending on local conditions.

Counselling is of paramount importance for any individual considering an HIV antibody test, as everyone contemplating taking a test is required to understand what they have agreed to, and the implications of any test result. This is known as *informed consent.* In order to give informed consent, it is therefore necessary to talk with a person who understands about HIV and its implications, and who is able to communicate that understanding to the person considering the issues. Many STD or GU clinics employ an HIV counsellor; additionally there are usually counsellors in the voluntary sector or in private practice. It is important that individuals should feel happy with their choice of counsellor and be able to opt for another counsellor if desired.

Testing at a GP surgery may at first appear more palatable than visiting a GU or STD clinic, but may have important drawbacks:

1. There may be little or no specialist counselling available at a GP surgery; and

2. A GP may be obliged to disclose details of medical records to insurance companies at a future date.

Whereas at a GU/STD clinic:

1. The NHS 1974 VD Regulations cover people attending GU and STD clinics and offers the tightest confidentiality in the NHS to those who attend;

2. The clinics usually refer to people by number, not by name. This can be checked out by telephone prior to a visit and may be less threatening to an individual; and

3. If a test is positive, the Communicable Disease Surveillance Centre in London, or Communicable Disease (Scotland) Unit, will be informed, but only for statistical reasons. They will be given the sex, age, county of testing and HIV status of the individual concerned, but no name or address. The clinic will not provide information to anyone else.

A person testing positive may wish to inform their GP from then on. They may want to ensure early medical help should the need arise and may feel that a good relationship with a GP is important for their psychological, as well as physical, wellbeing. Some people may wish to seek out a sympathetic GP and transfer to that practice before sharing their test result.

In some areas of Britain there are private clinics which may offer HIV counselling and testing. Whilst some would perhaps feel that standards of confidentiality and counselling may be better than those offered by the NHS, there is no reason to suppose that this is the case. Many NHS clinics now have wide experience of HIV issues and can offer a good service at no cost at all.

Table 3.10.1   Issues around where to go for counselling or testing

COUNSELLING ISSUES	GP	STD/GU CLINIC
Will my test result be kept totally confidential?	Yes. But may disclose to other doctors if it is in your best interest (medical intervention) or for the protection of others (e.g. spouse/partner)	Yes. Within NHS 1974 VD Regs, but if you are ill and need referring to a doctor within the hospital then it may go in medical hospital records.
	A GP may also have to disclose your result to an insurance company if you apply for life insurance	If your test is positive, the CDSC in London will be informed for statistical reasons only, your name will not be disclosed.
Will I be given adequate pre and post test counselling on all HIV issues?	Maybe, but most GP practices do not employ an HIV counsellor and may not have had enough experience of HIV themselves.	Yes, most clinics have excellent HIV counselling services, but you may like to 'shop around'.
Will I have to use my own name?	Yes.	No. It is not illegal to give a false name, but do remember it! In any case you may be given a number to use.

There is nothing to prevent a person who wishes to be conselled and tested in a different county to 'border hop'. Many people feel that little bit more in control by travelling to another city or county, and it is now generally accepted that this does happen. However, the grass may not always be greener in the next county and a telephone call to check on practice in another clinic could save a wasted journey.

Practitioners who have little experience of HIV counselling may find the chart (table 3.10.2) useful. It is aimed at counselling practice rather than session planning (see chapter 14).

Table 3.10.2 Counselling response

DO	DON'T
Listen;	Give advice;
Clarify any euphemisms e.g. 'having sex';	Minimise issues;
Correct any misinformation slowly and clearly;	Offer reassurance such as 'I'm sure you'll be alright', when you aren't sure at all;
Check out that the individual understands what you have said;	Hurry. Time is important to us all, but this cannot be rushed;
Ask for feedback or summary from the individual to clarify this;	Overload the individual with information;
Tell the individual how to get hold of you and when you are usually available; and	Make promises you can't keep, e.g. 'call me anytime';
Identify and reflect accurately emotions of the client throughout the session.	Work without adequate supervision; or
	Hand out leaflets about HIV as a substitute for discussion.

Preliminary counselling about HIV or AIDS issues

Those individuals attending a counselling session with concerns about HIV or AIDS will have certain needs in common which will have to be addressed by the counsellor. These include the individual's:

Understanding of HIV and AIDS;
Knowledge of HIV transmission;
Understanding of how HIV is not transmitted; and
Understanding of high/low risk practices.

Pretest counselling should ideally be in a second session *and there should be no expectation on the part of the counsellor that 'pretest' means that a test is inevitable.* An individual may well decide that a test is not for them and it is important that the counsellor does not behave as though it should be, just because the ground has been covered.

Table 3.10.3 may be of use to the counsellor when addressing pretest issues with those unsure about testing.

Table 3.10.3 Pretest issues

SOME REASONS FOR TESTING	SOME REASONS AGAINST TESTING
To take advantage of early medical help if test is positive.	If positive, insurance companies will not provide life cover.
When pregnant, or when considering becoming pregnant, as an HIV+ woman may pass the virus on to the baby.	If negative, individual may still have to answer further, personal, lifestyle questions and may still be refused cover or have premium increased.
To reduce the probability of infection and to enable the individual to lower anxiety to a manageable level.	Possible rejection by friends or partner if positive.
	Possible discrimination at work or with housing if positive.
	If test is positive, anxiety and stress levels may well be increased.
	A positive test may pose restrictions on entry to some countries.
THERE IS NO NEED TO HAVE A TEST IN ORDER TO ADOPT A SAFER LIFESTYE — i.e. safer sex, not sharing needles	

Post-test counselling must always be offered regardless of the test result. Listed in Table 3.10.4 are some possible outcomes and issues for the client and counsellor.

Table 3.10.4 Possible outcomes and issues for post test counselling

HIV+ RESULT	HIV− RESULT
Anxiety levels may be raised and there may be anger, tears and denial.	Relief which may be followed by reluctance to retest in 12 weeks time. May need follow-up session to discuss retest as a negative result should not be misunderstood.
Shock and fear.	
Blame (self or others).	
Guilt.	If this is the second negative result, then the individual will be relieved but will need to have safer lifestyle reinforced. May still need follow-up session.
Fear of isolation and rejection — who to share result with?	
Altered body image.	
Lack of interest in counsellor adressing safer lifestyle. Go sensitively and slowly.	
WHATEVER THE RESULT — OPTIONS FOR A SAFER LIFESTYLE SHOULD BE ADDRESSED — i.e. safer sex, not sharing needles	

11 Sociological issues

Safer sex

Safer sexual practice is sexual practice which reduces the likelihood of transmission of blood, semen or vaginal secretions, from one person to another. Good education around *safer sex* seeks to promote an understanding of risk activity in order that each individual can assess and reduce their risk of HIV infection and sexually transmitted diseases to an acceptable level. It has less to do with numbers of partners than with the resulting activity which may take place between those partners. (*See* chapter 9.) Personal belief or distaste about a particular sexual activity should never be substituted for truth when relating that practice to the risks of HIV infection, or other sexually transmitted diseases. Practitioners addressing aspects of safer sex need to be confident and comfortable with sexuality in general in order to be able to discuss them freely and openly with a child without fear or favour.

Children who have been coerced into sexual activities may find the idea of safer sex a difficult one to comprehend. It denotes choice and negotiation, and they have had neither. Young children will not be involved in a sexual relationship which is consensual, but will still need to understand what constitutes risky activity. Older children may be involved with boy or girlfriends (external to the abuse) and will want to know how they can avoid becoming infected or infecting others.

It is important that those working in this field communicate clearly with children using words which are understandable and honest. Euphemisms such as 'heavy petting' and 'sleeping with' are to be avoided as being unclear and imprecise. Practitioners need to establish early on with the child, a common language through which education can take place (*see* chapter 14) and be receptive to any new words the child wishes to use. Table 3.11.1 lists the most common sexual practices and how to reduce the risk of HIV transmission.

Table 3.11.1 Common sexual practices and how to reduce HIV transmission

ACTIVITY	RISK	HOW TO REDUCE RISK
Penetrative anal/ vaginal intercourse	HIGH in practice	Use condoms treated with NONOXYNOL 9® and plenty of water based lubricant, e.g. KY Jelly®.
Oral sex mouth/male sexual organs	MEDIUIM in theory*	Use dry or fruit flavoured condoms to avoid semen getting in contact with mouth lining.
Oral sex mouth/female sexual organs	MEDIUM in theory*	Avoid vaginal fluid or menstrual blood coming in contact with mouth lining. Use latex barrier such as dental dams.
Masturbation - self	NONE	
Masturbation - others	LOW	Make sure fingernails don't scratch inside of vagina/ anus causing bleeding. Fingerstalls or rubber gloves give added protection. Avoid getting semen into open cuts.
Kissing	NONE	There is no risk from saliva; only blood from bleeding gums.
Hugging, stroking, caressing	NONE	
Activity involving urine/faeces	NONE for HIV, but may be risk of Hepatitis B, salmonella or gut infections	Avoid getting urine/faeces in eyes or mouth. Wash out with plenty of cold water if this occurs.
Vibrators	LOW	Avoid sharing vibrators. Wash vibrator with hot soapy water after use.

*Whilst HIV transmission is theoretically possible in oral sex, there have been very few known cases.

Obviously some sexual practices here are less common than others but for those involved in working in the area of child sexual abuse, none will be new. It is important to point out the health hazards of some activities for the young person's future behaviour, whilst remembering their right to choice and options.

Some young people will ask for more detailed information than others and this chart should not be used as a list to work through with children. It is merely a reference for the practitioner, who will be able to judge what would and would not be helpful and appropriate in each circumstance. It can sometimes be useful to ask a young person to list as many sexual practices as they can think of, and place them in order of highest/lowest risk, using their new knowledge and perhaps the triangle of risk as a guide (*see* chapter 9). Provided that they have revealed all, it becomes plain when doing this how much has been understood and how it can be applied. It should also become clear that safer sexual practice is not just about condoms, but about alternatives to penetrative intercourse.

Young people involved in or contemplating consensual sexual relationships

Whilst condom usage can reduce the risk of HIV and other STDs substantially, there are perhaps three issues which need to be addressed before expecting that a knowledge of how HIV is transmitted can be translated into practice. They are, the availability of free condoms, the poor image of condoms in relation to romance and the skills of the young person to negotiate the use of condoms in a relationship.

Negotiating in sexual relationships is not just difficult for young people, it is difficult for many adults. A recent survey on sexual practice amongst the young in the South West of Britain highlights the fact that only one third of the people surveyed had used a condom during their last experience of sexual intercourse (Ford 1991). This has been interpreted with alarm by many newspapers and by some educators. Whilst recognising that this result certainly leaves a lot to be desired, it is perhaps more useful to concentrate media activity on acknowledging the fact that one third of young people *are* able not only to *buy* condoms, but actually *use* them. It would be interesting to know how many adults are able to say the same for themselves despite their relative maturity and awareness of STDs and HIV. Safer sexual practice is important for us all whatever our age. A concentrated effort is required to help people of all ages develop the skills required to ensure that knowledge about STDs can be applied to behaviour and to enable safer sexual practice to be viewed as the 'norm'.

The young person who has been involved in child sexual abuse will find negotiating and asserting very, very difficult. Role play can be useful in allowing a person to rehearse the skills required for such negotiations in a safe environment.

The following exercises (adapted from Aggleton 1990), can help address some of the factors involved in asserting and negotiating for safer sexual practice. Exercise one also highlights the imbalance of power which may occur in relationships.

Exercise one:

● Ask the person to list as many ways as they can think of to persuade a partner to take part in *any* sexual act, e.g.:
  'I only want to hold you';
  'I'll be very careful';
  'I love you — it'll be OK'.

Encourage as many ideas as possible and when the list is complete ask the young person to think of as many ways and reasons for saying 'NO'.

● Then repeat the exercise, this time making a list of ways to persuade a partner to take part in an *unsafe* sexual practice, e.g.:
  'You can't get pregnant the first time with a new partner';
  'It'll be safe if we stand up';
  'I'll marry you if anything happens';
  'Real men don't use condoms'.

Again, ask the young person to list ways and reasons for saying 'NO'.

● Ask if there was a difference between the first and second exercise.
● How did it feel to be saying 'NO' in:
  (a) Exercise one; and
  (b) Exercise two.
● How difficult would it be to say 'NO' in reality?
● Might they ever want to say 'YES'?
● How might they say 'YES' and still remain safe from STDs or HIV?
● Did they feel more in control as the persuader or the person saying 'NO'?
  What did they learn from that about relationships?

This exercise is powerful and liberating and is best done in an individual setting first. At a later stage it is useful to employ it in a group setting where young people can practice ways of replying to all statements during roleplay and experience saying 'NO' to a number of other young people. The peer group approach can throw up new strategies of challenging these statements and is a more realistic experience than in a one to one counselling session.

Another useful group method of practising negotiation is the merry-go-round method. It involves real issues and elicits helpful responses from peers. The size of the group is best at about eight.

Exercise two:

● Divide the group in two. Sit one half of the group in a circle on chairs facing outwards. Place a chair which is empty in front of each 'listener'. Ask the remaining young people to think of a relationship situation with which they would have most difficulty coping. Ask them to sit on a chair facing a 'listener' and explain their problem. The helper must listen and then try and help formulate a response which would be useful to the person presenting the situation. Allow about five minutes before asking everyone in the outside circle to move one chair to the right. They then repeat the question until they have asked all the 'listeners'.

● Repeat the exercise with the 'listeners' now becoming the ones asking for help.

● Allow about 20–30 minutes to 'debrief'.

● Was the response of the 'listeners' useful?
 If so, why?
 If not, why not?
 Are there any situations with which people still need some help?

This exercise provides a forum for solving or managing real issues which may have been the worst possible 'what if' scenario in the young person's head. Not all issues can be solved, but many can be managed better if the skills are in that young persons 'tool kit'. This exercise will also highlight areas where more work needs to be done. Two counsellors are a **must** for this exercise as it can cause abreaction of emotion and is a 'later stage' rather than a 'first stage' exercise.

Condom usage

A young person asking about condom usage should be shown how to use a condom safely. Most AIDS educators/counsellors are skilled in demonstrating condom usage without embarrassment and take care to stress the positive health messages in relation to STDs. Those who are new to condom demonstration may find Table 3.11.2 useful when teaching.

Addressing and dealing with issues of safer sexual practice may limit the future risks to that individual. Recent research in the US shows that females who have experienced sexual abuse in childhood are nearly three times as likely to become pregnant by the age of 18. Males who experienced childhood sexual abuse have a twofold increase in HIV prevalence. Both males and females who experienced childhood sexual abuse were four times more likely to be involved in prostitution (Zierler et al 1991).

The report concluded that early identification of victims of child sexual abuse may be important in managing HIV risk factors in the future. If this is indeed the case, educators should not shy away from attempting to teach children who have experienced child sexual abuse about safer sex, but should work together with relevant agencies to offer assistance where needed.

Life insurance — the present problem

Life insurance is offered at the discretion of the insurer and is not an automatic right. Whilst the advertisements portray an image of all caring altruism, life insurance companies are in the business of making profits, and as such go to great lengths to minimise losses in revenue by assessing the risk to themselves, by means of an applicant questionnaire or proposal form.

One of the questions which an applicant is likely to be asked deals directly with HIV/AIDS. The applicant may be asked if they have ever had a test or counselling for HIV infection. If the answer to this is 'yes', then the insurer will ask why this took place and will ask for the result of the test. If the result of the test was positive then life insurance will be refused. Should this happen then an applicant's name is entered on the Impaired Lives Register by the insurance company, and other insurance companies who have access to the register will also refuse the applicant ordinary life insurance. This register is for serious medical conditions where lives are uninsurable.

The child who has experienced child sexual abuse and received counselling or undergone HIV testing is likely to view insurance as a vague and distant problem which has little significance to the present day. It is important however, to explain the present position with regard to insurance to a child or parent, despite the fact that this

Table 3.11.2   Condom usage demonstration

STAGES	TEACHING POINTS
Prepare equipment	Explain the use of penis-substitute (carrot) and why its use adds humour and dispels any embarrassment
Look at packet of condoms	Check that packet has a kitemark, check sell-by date, check whether spermicide is used as a lubricant (Nonoxynol 9)
Take one condom from packet	Check to see that foil is not damaged
Open foil wrapper carefully Remove condom from wrapper	Make sure fingernails or rings don't catch or tear contents
Place condom in palm of hand and allow young person to look at it	Young people may never have seen a condom before
Place thumb inside condom and gently push teat so it stands up	Explain that teat is a vital part of condom, and is a receptacle for sperm
Gently squeeze teat between finger and thumb to expel air	Explain that when ejaculation takes place pressure is put on end of condom, and condom may split if air is not expelled before using
Place condom on end of carrot	Explain that penis must be erect before condom is used
Unroll condom down length of carrot	Explain that condom must be put on before penis comes into contact with partner, as pre-ejaculation fluid can sometimes leak out prior to intercourse
Penetration can now take place	Explain that if more lubricant is needed then a water based gel should be used, as oil based gels destroy rubber
After ejaculation, hold condom in place and withdraw	Explain that it is important to withdraw before the penis goes limp to avoid danger of semen leaking from top of condom
Remove condom and tie a knot in it	Explain that this contains the semen and reduces the risk of spillage when discarding it
Place condom in a tissue and put in a rubbish bin	Explain that condoms are not biodegradable and pollution is irresponsible

position may change in the coming years. Informed consent to testing assumes an understanding of today's facts rather than tomorrow's speculation, and the practitioner should not ignore this issue simply because practices in insurance companies may have changed by the time the child becomes an adult.

Questions about insurance and mortgages which children may routinely ask:

What is life insurance?
Life insurance is an agreement between you and an insurance company. You pay the insurance company a small amount of money each month and, in return, if you die before a certain date, the company will pay a large amount of money to your partner or children.

What is a mortgage?
A mortgage is an agreement between you and whoever lends you money to buy a house. In return for lending you the money they have certain rights to that house until all the money plus interest is paid back. Some people borrow money for just 10 years, but others may borrow money for up to 30 years.

Why would I need life insurance to get a mortgage?
You wouldn't always *need* it, there are ways of getting a mortgage without it, but you may *want* it. If you died before you could pay back the money you owed for the house, then the life insurance money would pay back all that you owed. Your partner or children would not have to worry about how to pay to keep the house.

Why would an insurance company want to know if I have had an HIV test?
They would want to know how likely it wold be that you were at risk from something that might mean you would die earlier than expected.

Why?
Because if you were HIV positive, they would think that there would be more chance of having to pay out a large amount of money before the date on the agreement.

Have I got to tell the insurance company if I have a test?
Yes, you need to be truthful when you fill in the form.

What happens if I lie?
If you lie and the insurance company find out, you will find that your agreement with the company is cancelled and you will lose all the money you paid in and get nothing back.

If the test is negative, will I get insurance?
Yes, you should, providing that the insurance company is happy with
the reason why you had a test, and providing that there are no other
things happening in your life that they would think were risky. You
would need to get advice from experts who would help find the best
policy for you.

Where would I find an expert?
If you contacted the Terrence Higgins Trust in London (telephone:
071-831-0330) they would put you in touch with the right people to
help you.

If my test is positive will I be able to get life insurance?
No, you will not be able to get ordinary life insurance but you may be
able to get a policy that pays out for death caused by something other
than an AIDS related illness.

So if I were positive could I still buy a house?
Yes, you can buy a house without life insurance. The person giving you
a mortgage can sometimes arrange a mortgage known as a repayment
mortgage, or you can apply for an interest only mortgage. The
Terrence Higgins Trust can advise on whom to contact for the best plan
for you.

Travelling abroad

Despite the fact that most countries in the world have some cases of
HIV infection, the general attitude in many countries appears to be one
which denies a pre-existence of HIV infection and assumes that HIV
comes from elsewhere, brought in by tourists and immigrants. To this
end, many countries have introduced discriminatory measures ranging
from compulsory HIV testing on arrival at borders, to deportation if
discovered to be HIV positive. Neither action is supported by the
Council of Europe (1987) or by the World Health Organisation (1987)
who state respectively that these actions are ethically and scientifically
unjustifiable and that no screening programme is able to prevent the
introduction and spread of HIV infection into any country.
    As travel restrictions for those with HIV infection may alter, it is
perhaps worth checking with the appropriate diplomatic agency of a
country before making plans for holidays or travel. Aggleton maintains
'It should be recognised, however, that discrepancies can often arise
between the stated policy of a government, and the practices of its
border and immigration officials' (Aggleton et al 1989). Therefore, a

telephone call to the British Red Cross may give access to a more complete picture of any restrictions in any particular country at any given time.

A child's doctor should also be consulted prior to travel abroad with reference to the child receiving appropriate vaccine in the light of their HIV status.

Holiday insurance

Families with children who are HIV positive and who want to travel abroad, should look carefully at clauses in holiday insurance proposals before assuming that any HIV related claim, whilst abroad, would be met.

Some policies operate a simple HIV/AIDS exclusion clause, but other policies have clauses which may be less obvious at first glance, but which may refuse cover 'for any illness directly or indirectly attributable to a sexually transmitted disease' or for 'non-disclosure of chronic medical conditions'.

This is not to say that it is impossible to obtain health insurance whilst travelling. As with all forms of insurance there will always be cover available providing the applicant can afford the increased premium.

It may be possible to obtain insurance with perhaps a slightly increased premium simply by asking the consultant or paediatrician for a letter confirming the child's fitness to travel. Many EC countries operate reciprocal arrangements for health care and for those wishing to travel in Europe, an E111 form, available from any DSS office, should be completed prior to leaving the UK. Even without an E111, those travelling in Europe can obtain emergency health care by paying for it at the time and claiming reimbursement on arrival home.

References and Resources

Aggleton P, Homans H, Mojsa J, Watson S, Watney S, 1989 *AIDS: scientific and social issues*. Churchill Livingstone.

Aggleton P, Horsley C, Warwick I, Wilton T, 1990 *AIDS working with young people*. AVERT.

British Red Cross Society, London, 9 Grosvenor Crescent, London, SW1X 7EJ. Telephone: 071-235 5454.

Council of Europe 1987 Recommendation R(87)25.

Ford, 1991 The sexual behaviour of young people and directions for the promotion of safer sex. *Royal Society of Medicine AIDS Letter* No 27.

Terrence Higgins Trust. 52-54 Grays Inn Road, London, WC1X 8JU. Telephone: 071-831 0330.

WHO, 1987 *Report of the consultative committee on international travel and HIV 2 infection.*

Zeirler et al, May 1991 Adult survivors of childhood sexual abuse and subsequent risk of HIV infection. *American Journal of Public Health* **81**(5).

12 Legal and ethical aspects of AIDS

First do no harm

Today's limited research shows that a positive antibody test, in children who have been sexually abused, is relatively uncommon.

In approximately 1,000 tests in the US, on victims of sexual abuse, only two were found to be HIV positive (Gellert 1990). Neither victim had been assessed for other risk factors and it is not known whether they were HIV positive prior to the abuse taking place (Fost 1990).

Elsewhere in the US, over a two year period, a paediatric team saw 96 children who were HIV positive. Fourteen of these children had been sexually abused, but only four were proved to have contracted HIV through sexual abuse (Gutman et al 1991).

Whilst, theoretically, every instance of unprotected penetrative intercourse can be seen as a potential HIV risk, to adopt HIV antibody testing, on a widespread basis, for all children who have been sexually abused may be seen as an abuse in itself (Honigsbaum 1991). It may do further harm to the child in terms of unnecessary worry. Testing should only be offered when it becomes an issue for the child, or parent, or when it can be shown that the future health of the child would be at risk without such intervention. Even then a test should only take place after educative/counselling sessions and with the *informed consent* either of the child, if of sufficient understanding, or of a person with parental responsibility. The General Medical Council stated in 1988 that:

> 'It has long been accepted, and is well understood within the profession, that a doctor should treat a patient only on the basis of the patient's informed consent'.

However, it then went on to differentiate the circumstances required for implicit and explicit consent:

'A patient's consent may in certain circumstances be given implicitly, for example by agreement to provide a specimen of blood for multiple analysis. *In other circumstances it needs to be given explicitly, for example before undergoing a specified operative procedure or providing a specimen of blood to be tested specifically for a named condition.*'

It can be clearly seen from my emphasis in the last sentence, that blood sampling for an antibody test falls into the need for explicit consent. The GMC recognises that simply *having* an antibody test can have serious consequences for an individual both financially and socially. It argues that each patient be given advance opportunity to assess the implications of any such test prior to accepting or declining it. They go on to state that:

'Only in the most exceptional circumstances, where a test is imperative in order to secure the safety of persons other than the patient, and where it is not possible for the prior consent of the patient to be obtained, can testing without explicit consent be justified'.

Failure to obtain consent may result in an action against the doctor for negligence, as the doctor is required to explain the purpose of any implications of treatment. However, to what extent the doctor explains the proposed action and consequences of treatment still remains a question of individual clinical judgement. Should the doctor decide to exercise his/her discretion and test for antibodies without the specific consent of the individual and without clinical grounds, then that doctor would have to be prepared to justify that action to both the GMC and the law courts (BMA 1988).

Should the perpetrator be tested?

It may be felt that it would be more appropriate to test the perpetrator of the sexual abuse rather than the child. Extreme caution needs to be taken if considering this option, as it may be more of a panic reaction on the part of the professional, rather than a well thought out sensible move. Whilst it could be argued that the test was imperative to secure the safety of persons other than the individual (*see* above), consideration should also be given to the rights of the individual, and to the possible outcomes of testing for that individual. It may be difficult to listen to the small sweet voice of reason when dealing with this emotive issue, but clear thinking needs to be in place in order to justify this as a rational rather than merely punitive action. It would be necessary to obtain consent from the perpetrator prior to testing, and to offer adequate pretest counselling and support. If consent is refused and a test is carried out, such action will be a breach of the duty of care and actionable in negligence. However, as d'Eca maintains 'the difficulty in such an action will be proving damage and quantifying any loss' (d'Eca 1990).

Should consent be refused, a medical practitioner may apply to a magistrate for an order for medical examination in accordance with Section 38 of the Public Health (Infectious Diseases) Regulations 1985. If a magistrate issues such an order and examination is carried out despite repeated refusal to consent, such action will be an assault on the individual and the medical practitioner may be required to justify this action in court (d'Eca 1990). This is because there is no provision in the legislation for dispensing with consent to treatment. Failure to comply with an order for medical examination results only in a fine.

Perpetrators who test positive may have infected their victim(s), but equally may have contracted the virus after the last incidence of abuse. The victim(s) may or may not be infected with HIV and may or may not decide to be tested themselves.

Perpetrators who test negative may not be infected with HIV but, as explained in chapter 10, false negatives do occur. The uncertainty remains the same for the victims, who will still need to decide for themselves whether or not to be tested.

In short, either result will still raise the same uncertainties about testing victims and is of no advantage, although a perpetrator who tests positive will obviously cause added concern to all involved. Perpetrators of sexual abuse who know themselves to be HIV positive at the time of the abuse, and who have infected their victim, may be liable to heavier sentencing by the courts. There may also be justification for a higher Criminal Injuries Compensation Board (CICB) award to the victim. If the perpetrator is dead, consent for blood sampling will need to be obtained from next of kin. However, it cannot be stressed too strongly that in testing a perpetrator, alive or dead, the issue for the victim remains one of uncertainty.

Is a child able to consent?

The ability of a child to understand and give consent to antibody testing depends on each individual child. The GMC make provision for this in their guidelines:

> 'A particular difficulty arises in cases where it may be desirable to test a child for HIV infection and where, consequently, the consent of a parent, or a person in loco parentis, would normally be sought. However, the possibility that the child may have been infected by a parent may, in

certain circumstances, distort the parent's judgement so that consent is withheld in order to protect the parent's own position. The doctor faced with this situation must first judge whether the child is competent to consent to the test on his or her own behalf. If the child is judged competent in this context, then consent can be sought from the child. If however the child is judged unable to give consent the doctor must decide whether the interests of the child should override the wishes of the parent. It is the view of the Council that it would not be unethical for a doctor to perform such a test without parental consent, provided always that the doctor is able to justify that action as being in the best interests of the patient.'

It is more straightforward for the practitioner if parental/guardian consent can be obtained prior to testing, but in many instances this is not appropriate, and children may be asked to make that decision themselves. This is supported by the Law Lords ruling that:

'at common law, children and young people have the capacity to make decisions for themselves on matters which affect them, if capable of understanding the issues, and of making up their own minds on the matter requiring decision' (Children's Legal Centre).

Alternatively, a specific issue order could be sought under Section 8 of the 1989 *Children Act.*

The judgement in the Gillick case expressly mentions younger children and states that children under 16 hold an independent right to consent or withhold consent if 'they have sufficient understanding and intelligence to make the decision' (Scarman 1985). However, it remains to be seen what attitude the courts will take to the decision in Gillick when dealing with applications concerning children under Section 8 of the *Children Act.*

The implications for the practitioner involve assessing the ability of the child to understand the nature of the test and its repercussions. This is addressed more fully in chapter 13.

Confidentiality and public interest

All professionals will be bound by their employers' code of confidentiality and by their professional guidelines. These codes may vary slightly from profession to profession but exist for the protection of the client (and in some cases, the employer), whilst reinforcing the integrity of the professional.

Codes and guidelines do not supplant the law however, and individuals are also obliged to keep confidential all information which they receive in a trusting relationship (Harris 1990). This is the law or obligation of confidence, and can be applied to organisational relationships or even friendships. Only if a court is convinced that disclosure of confidential information is in the public interest can there be justification for breaching confidence. It is important when dealing with HIV issues to recognise the difference between those professionals who 'need to know' and those who would 'like to know' when a child/parent/perpetrator may be considering antibody testing. Human nature, being what it is, thrives on speculation and drama. There will therefore, be a need for responsible recording of information and some interagency understanding of rights of access to information as this may vary in each profession. Department of Health guidelines state:

> 'Staff in different agencies, and other practitioners, will maintain their own records of the case and such records should be subject to the arrangements for maintaining confidentiality within that particular agency. Well kept records are essential to good child protection practice and each agency should have a policy stating the purpose and the format for keeping records; this should cover the need to retain records for appropriate periods. All agencies must establish procedures to safeguard information provided to them and to ensure timely transfer of relevant records when a child and/or family moves to or from an area'.
>
> (Department of Health 1991).

Despite this sensible advice it could, and may, be argued that it would not be in the best interests of the child to disclose to others that HIV counselling or testing has taken place. If the child asks that this is kept confidential then counsellors may refuse to give this information on request, and remain within the law, until they are instructed by a court of law to disclose such information.

Counsellors who experience a conflict over the sharing of information received from the child should follow the following guidelines:

> 'In child protection work the degree of confidentiality will be governed by the need to protect the child. Social workers and others working with a child and family must make clear to those providing information that *confidentiality may not be maintained if the withholding of the information will prejudice the welfare of a child.* Department of Health guidance to social services departments on the confidentiality and disclosure of personal information is contained in LAC(88)17 'Personal Social Services: Confidentiality of Personal Information'.
>
> (Department of Health 1991).

My italics highlight the need for counsellors to recognise when breaking a child's confidence may be in the best interests of the child, and act accordingly, being prepared to justify their conduct.

The Children's Legal Centre maintain that: 'At the very least children have a right to know in what circumstances confidentiality may not be respected' (Childrens Legal Centre). Even the knowledge that an individual has had an HIV antibody test, can have far reaching social consequences for that individual in the future. Confidential record keeping is of paramount importance, and policies for such recording should be established, if not already in place.

Where to get legal advice on AIDS issues

Legal issues around AIDS and HIV can be complex and specialist help should be sought if in doubt about a course of action. Some sources of good legal advice include:

The Terrence Higgins Trust (THT)
Legal, Welfare Rights Centre
52-54 Grays Inn Road
London WC1X 8JU
Tel: 071-831 0330

THT advice centre offers legal, welfare rights and housing advice. It has a solicitor, two welfare rights workers, a housing officer and administrative support. THT's current solicitor has particular interest in child care law and gives advice on all aspects of HIV.
Home and hospital visits are undertaken.
THT have published 'AIDS: A Guide to the Law' edited by Dai Harris and Richard Haigh. Available from the THT.

Immunity
260a Kilburn Lane
London W10 4BA
Tel: 081-968 8909

Legal Advice and Representation and Welfare Rights.
This is the UK's first established legal centre to help people address legal and welfare issues around HIV and AIDS.
Two lawyers give free legal advice to those with a London home address on HIV/AIDS problems. Telephone advice is also available for those who live elsewhere.
There is a home or hospital visiting service, but most people visit the Immunity office for appointments with lawyers.
Immunity have produced a good series of leaflets on legal rights.

Immunity and Terrence Higgins Trust have established a good working relationship and are recognised as centres of excellence.

Children's Legal Centre
20 Compton Terrace
London N1 2UN
Tel: 071-359 9392

The Children's Legal Centre produces a range of excellent information sheets and booklets on all aspects of children and the law.

National AIDS Manual (NAM)
NAM Publications Ltd
Unit 136 Brixton Enterprise Centre
444 Brixton Road
London SW9 8EJ
Tel: 071-737 1846

This is a good reference manual dealing with medical, social and legal issues. It contains addresses of all agencies dealing with aspects of HIV/AIDS and updates are mailed to subscribers regularly.

References

BMA Conference, 1988.

Children and confidentiality — the legal position. Children's Legal Centre.

Children's Legal Centre *Landmark decision for Children's Rights.* Information sheet.

d'ECA, 1990 Medicolegal Aspects of AIDS. *AIDS a guide to the law,* Harris and Haigh. (eds) Tavistock/Routledge.

Department of Health 1991 *Working Together Under the Children Act 1989* para 3.16 p13. Reproduced with permission of Her Majesty's Stationery Office.

Fost, 1990 Ethical Considerations in Testing Victims of Sexual Abuse for HIV infection. *Child Abuse and Neglect* **14**: 5–7.

Gellert, 1990 Developing Guidelines for HIV antibody testing among victims of paediatric sexual abuse. *Child abuse and neglect* **14**: 9–17.

Gillick v West Norfolk and Wisbech Area Health Authority (1985).

Gutman L T et al, 1991 *American journal of diseases of children* **145**(2): 137–41.

Harris, 1990 AIDS and employment. *AIDS a guide to the law*. Harris and Haigh (eds). Tavistock/Routledge.

Honigsbaum, 1991 *HIV/AIDS and children*. National Children's Bureau.

Lord Scarman, 1985 House of Lords. 3 All ER 402.

Section 35, 61 Public Health (Infectious Diseases) Regs 1985.

13 Issues to be addressed when planning guidelines for HIV/AIDS counselling in child sexual abuse

Why counsel at all?

It has been strongly recommended that HIV antibody testing should only take place after informed consent has been obtained from the individual. The GMC also recommend that consensual testing should only take place after pretest counselling has been given.

Children and adults have a right to know and understand the limitations of an antibody test and to recognise what social restrictions may be levied against them should it be known that testing has taken place, e.g. difficulty with travel and insurance. The child also needs to be aware of the advantages in having a test in terms of medical intervention for prophylactic treatment. Children need time to discuss any worries they may have about HIV/AIDS. Many children today will have received some information from the media on this issue, and it is wise to check that this received wisdom is in fact correct and fully understood by the child. Parents/guardians of abused children frequently have HIV concerns and it is important to offer counselling in order that informed choices can be made. Nobody would pretend that counselling will always eradicate the issue, but it may help a child/parent manage that issue more effectively.

Who should counsel?

Many professionals and workers in the voluntary sector use counselling skills in helping people manage their lives more effectively. In the field of child sexual abuse there are many skilled practitioners who are able to deal sensitively and productively with the physical, emotional and psychological effects of sexual abuse. These may include:

- Doctors
- Psychologists
- Psychiatrists
- Social workers
- Health advisers/educators

AIDS/HIV issues may pose special problems for those who counsel in that:

- Conflicting information or grey areas exist
- No cure for HIV infection or AIDS exists at present
- HIV is infectious for life
- People with HIV infection may become stigmatised and isolated

Rather than attempt to define which discipline is best suited to counsel in this area, it is perhaps more important to list what would be useful background experience or skills for anyone considering this role. These could include:

- Proven counselling skills with in-depth experience of one or more counselling model
- Knowledge and understanding of human sexuality and sexual response
- Good communication skills, verbal and non verbal
- Ability to relate to young people on equal terms
- Assertion and negotiating skills
- Knowledge of child developmental issues
- Understanding of the issue of power in sexual relationships including child sexual abuse
- Understanding of different health promotion models in relation to behavioural outcome
- Experience in psychotherapeutic counselling skills

- Experience in participatory approaches in working with children and adults and AIDS/HIV
- Evaluation skills
- Commitment to personal development in relation to sexuality and prejudice

The importance of the last requirement cannot be stressed too strongly. If a counsellor has unresolved issues about sexuality they may all too easily be triggered off in a counselling setting. The place for such issues to be addressed and resolved is in a personal development setting and never during a counselling/educative session with a client.

Counsellors should also demonstrate a non-judgemental attitude and have a warm, honest and committed approach.

Who makes referrals for counselling?

A recognised referral system is an integral part of any framework for providing HIV counselling. It is necessary to assess who is the most appropriate person to accept referrals and plan accordingly. These referrals may be made directly by the doctor responsible for the medical examination of the child, or via that medical department from social workers, teachers, GPs, psychologists etc. It is advisable that referrals are in writing and that adequate provision is provided for the confidential nature of written referrals. It may also be advisable that any telephone referrals made to a counsellor by the referee should be followed by a covering letter which could include details of parental or other consent to counselling. Some though may also need to be given to the safe-keeping of notes, if any, made by the counsellor (*see* chapter 12).

Who should be present at the counselling session?

Guidelines may also need to focus on whether a child should see a counsellor alone or be accompanied by an appropriate adult. Consideration should be given to the child's age, understanding and wishes. An accompanying adult may help a child feel secure, or may be a barrier to honest communications. In some instances it may be more appropriate to counsel a parent or guardian, in the case of children under the age of seven years, or those who are not of sufficient understanding and intelligence to receive benefit from such counselling.

Supervision and support

Whilst facilitating training in multiagency settings, it has become apparent that there is some confusion and discrepancy between counselling supervision/support, and basic line management supervision/support. This confusion is also commented on in the British Association for Counselling (BAC) *HIV Counselling Report* 1990, which recommends the following:

1. A combined system of supervision by line management and independent counselling supervision/consultative support is recommended for all HIV counsellors.
2. It is recommended that the cost of providing this system of supervision in terms of time and any fees paid should normally be the agency's   responsibility.
3. Agencies who are funding the independent counselling/consultative support should be actively involved in establishing a clear contract between the HIV counsellor, line management and independent counselling supervision/consultative support which identifies the responsibility of each to the others.
4. Further research should be undertaken to review the implementation of these recommendations and develop more detailed recommendations about the good practice of the supervision of HIV counsellors.

Members of BAC who practice are required to have supervision and support in accordance with the *Code of Ethics and Practice for Counsellors* (1990): 'It is a breach of the ethical requirement for counsellors to practise without regular counselling supervision/ consultative support'.

However, there are counsellors who have had to pay privately for counselling supervision as none has been provided by their employer, other than line management. Additionally there are others whose line managers do not understand the principles of supervision and feel that those who request it are somehow being weak or unprofessional.

Whatever the professional background of the practitioner, given the stress and personal issues which may surface when dealing with:

(a)   HIV counselling; and
(b)   child sexual abuse;

as well as the need to evaluate good practice, nobody should be expected to counsel on HIV issues in sexual abuse unless adequate supervision and support is provided. Supervision should be seen as an integral part of the counselling process and is an entitlement, not a privilege.

The flowchart in Figure 3.13.1 looks at possible provision of services to those requesting HIV counselling, and their carers. Those involved in using counselling skills or acting in formal counselling sessions need to recognise their limitations and refer on where and when appropriate, e.g. medical interventions.

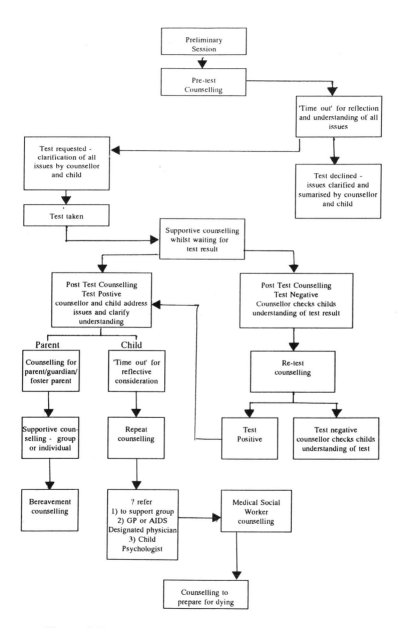

Figure 3.13.1   Flowchart for HIV counselling services

References

BAC, 1990 *Code of Ethics and Practice for Counsellors.*

Bond, 1990 *HIV counselling report on national survey and consultation.*
BAC/DoH.

14 Planning and implementing the counselling session

Initial responses

Children may ask about AIDS at any time during the course of the investigation and not always in the most appropriate settings. For a practitioner lacking the factual knowledge needed, the planned response could be:

'I don't know the answer to that would you like me to find out?'
'I don't know the answer to that would you like me to find someone who does?'
'I don't know the answer to that shall we find out together?'

It is far better to admit uncertainty than to guess at the answer in an attempt to allay fears. However, if it is simply that the question is asked in an inappropriate place, such as a corridor, then it may be useful to say 'Shall we go and find somewhere a bit quieter where we can talk?' The ideal discussion of course, will take place in a planned counselling session.

Where should it take place?

When giving consideration to a venue in which to meet the child the following points may need to be checked:

How near is it to where the child lives?
Is the venue comfortable and quiet?

Can you be overheard?
Does it offer easy, discreet access?
Is the venue intimidating?
How near is the washroom/lavatory?
Are there facilities for making drinks?
Is there a waiting area for parent/guardian/social worker?

Some practitioners may find that their own office fulfils all the criteria. Others will be sharing busy offices with little or no privacy, and certainly not all offices are appropriate. They may leave a lot to be desired in terms of interruptions, in person or by telephone; or in decor. A desk can be intimidating and can be a barrier to effective communication.

Many towns now have child and family centres which have rooms designed for comfort and which may fulfil all the necessary requirements. These can usually be booked in advance through Social Services and are far less threatening to the child than a clinic or hospital setting.

Some community centres, community schools, and social services departments can also be useful resources when considering where to hold a meeting.

Some practitioners may feel it would be most appropriate to see a child at home. If this is a possible option, do remember that it may not always be possible to control telephone interruptions, television or barking dogs, and perhaps may be best avoided.

Is it education or counselling?

Specialist counselling has both an educative and therapeutic element. The child/parent expects to be able to ask direct questions about HIV/AIDS of the practitioner and to receive direct answers. They may also expect to receive advice. Advice however, should not be on the agenda for the practitioner, who instead should offer a range of information from which an informed choice for action can be made by the child/parent, after consideration of all options. As Egan (1990) maintains 'Learning takes place when options are increased'.

The therapeutic element in AIDS counselling is directly related to the options chosen by the child/parent around HIV/AIDS issues such as testing, safer sex etc, and the feelings these arouse. The practitioner is not there to deal with specialist child abuse counselling and although there is frequently an overlap from one issue to the other, it is important that practitioners recognise their limitations and take advantage of specialist help and refer on as soon as it becomes necessary, e.g. to child psychologist or psychiatrist.

Similarly the practitioner may refer the child/parent for specialist medical help when it becomes apparent that advice on medical interventions is required.

An AIDS counselling session differs from an AIDS education session mainly in that counselling skills rather than teaching skills are used to inform and evaluate. Having said that, there will always be an overlap in education and counselling about AIDS as most educators and counsellors are aware. An understanding of both is important for a clear overview and a balanced perspective.

Counselling in individual or group settings?

By its very nature of being a confidential relationship, counselling should ideally take place on an individual basis, so that children have the opportunity to discuss all their concerns about HIV infection.

Those with experience in work with child sexual abuse will know that a child may perhaps disclose only one third of the extent of the abuse to social workers, police or those making the referral. Children may hold information back for a variety of reasons, the most common in my experience being the fear of 'being thought badly of'. The hidden part of the iceberg may never come to light or may well surface in HIV counselling when a child has deep concerns for their wellbeing. There is a strong chance, therefore, that the counsellor may get to hear more of the story than anyone else and should never assume that a referral which, in good faith, identifies low risk activity, is a complete picture of what really happened.

In terms of being able to assess HIV risk as accurately as possible, this 'hidden agenda' is very important. The counsellor should therefore be aware that the child's story may change during the course of the counselling and that the full story, or the amount of information that a child may wish to share with a counsellor, depends much upon the level of trust which a child develops for that counsellor.

It is highly unlikely that any new information will be disclosed if the counselling/educative session is in a group setting with more than one child. Children involved in multiple or familial abuse may have an agreement, implicit or explicit, to stick to the same story. They are skilled at keeping secrets and their allegiance will remain with the group story even when the counsellor has a very strong feeling that the level of concern about HIV infection seems to outweigh the disclosed 'low risk activity'. Peer group learning has great value and can take place alongside any counselling but it is important not to confuse the two issues, or to move too quickly to a group setting before addressing individual concerns in private. The counsellor is there for the child's interests, a conviction of the perpetrator is not enough. The needs of the child outweigh the sentence. We must be certain that a child has the opportunity to disclose as an individual, what they may not disclose in a group, about risk activity.

Who should be present?

If the child is under the age of seven, then a person acting in a parental role should be present. However, it may be far more appropriate to counsel the parent/guardian of a child so young, rather than the child itself, *unless the child is asking questions directly related to AIDS/HIV.* These days many children already have some knowledge of AIDS/ HIV from the media and from peers. They have a right to discuss those ideas and share their fears about possible infection.

Children over the age of seven may like a parent/guardian or social worker to be present and should be given this option. A child also needs to understand that they have control over the meeting and that they can ask the third party to leave the room at any time. A practitioner sensing hesitation part-way through a session should be sensitive to the situation and ask if the child would rather the third party left the room.

If a third party does attend a session, their role needs to be clarified at the start of the meeting, as some practitioners may expect the companion to remain silent but supportive, rather than be a vocal contributor to the meeting.

What is needed for the meeting?

Once the venue has been arranged it is important to decide what may be needed to facilitate a useful session with the child. I always take along a large pad of flipchart paper and some big felt tip markers. Although I have never taken reference books into a session, I see no reason why a practitioner should not do this if they will be useful. It does no harm to say 'I'm not sure about that — shall we look it up in this book?' Recently I have begun to take fresh orange juice and doughnuts, biscuits or fruit into a session which may last more than an hour. This may have a double benefit of introducing informality around a makeshift picnic, as well as being a good reason for having brought a box of tissues along. Tissues alone on a table can raise anxieties about crying. Tissues on which to wipe sticky fingers can also be used for tears, but do not raise the feeling that crying is an expectation.

There is a place for humour in the counselling session and applied sensitively, it has a great role in diffusing tension and anxiety.

How to start a session

In the context of HIV counselling, the issue of child sexual abuse can sometimes be more of an emotional 'red herring' for the counsellor than it is for the child *at that moment.*

In other words the issue for the child is more likely to be HIV/AIDS than it is to be the sexual abuse, which should be being dealt with by a psychiatrist/psychologist, or specially trained social worker.

This has been the case in all sessions I have experienced with children whether the abuse stems from a paedophile ring or is familial. Sexual abuse is on the child's agenda but, during the session, AIDS is higher up. This statement is not intended to belittle the child's experience of sexual abuse, but rather to put it in the context of HIV counselling, so that the practitioner can see that they are dealing with the possibility of risk activity in relation to HIV, not in relation to child sexual abuse. That is for other sessions with, perhaps, other professionals.

It is important to start a session with a child by saying who you are and what you are there for. Clarification of the role of the third party is also important at this stage. A simple statement about how confidentiality is applied can also be made now (*see* chapter 12). It is important to tell the child in what circumstances you may have a duty to share information with somebody else.

Tell the child how long the session will last. It may be an hour or you may have planned a lot longer. Whatever you plan, it is important to indicate the timescale at the start.

After all this you are ready to begin and a useful question may be 'What has made you want to see me today?' or even simpler 'How can I help you?' Gentle, open questions can encourage the child to define their main concern about AIDS and the following checklist may be useful for a preliminary meeting:

CHECKLIST FOR PRELIMINARY COUNSELLING SESSION	
What is the main concern of the child at the present time?	Listen carefully and don't be tempted to minimise issue or offer reassurance or platitudes.
What do they understand by HIV and AIDS?	Clarify and correct information where necessary.

What do they know about how HIV is passed on?	Clarify and correct, check out any euphemisms i.e. through sex/sleeping together 'What does child mean by sex/ sleeping together'?
How many activities can they think of in which HIV is not passed on?	Clarify and correct. Check level of existing knowledge.
Can they tell you how they think they may have become infected with HIV?	Clarify and identify any risk activity.

Communicating with the child

The language that is used throughout the session should be one that is understood clearly by the child and the practitioner. Children are unlikely to use words like penis, vagina, anus, and penetrative intercourse. They will have their own words for these and you will need to find out what they are.

A simple but effective exercise can be to draw a rough outline of a man or woman and ask the child to tell you what words they would use for different parts of the body. Explain to the child that you need to be able to understand each other and that people use many different words for the same thing. It then becomes easy to say 'I use these words, some people use these other words — what words do you use?'. If a particularly puzzling word crops up in a session it can be clarified by the practitioner saying 'That's an interesting/funny word, can you tell me what it means?'. Many new words may be learned in such meetings and most will be much more 'user friendly' than the medical equivalents. Check also what words the child uses for semen and vaginal fluid. In terms of risk activity this is very important, after all, a 'snake which spits' or a 'mousie being sick' are very different ways to describe a penis ejaculating semen.

What may happen during a session?

It is difficult to generalise about the outcome of the meeting. Table 3.14.1 lists possible outcomes with some pointers for what may be useful responses.

Table 3.14.1 Possible outcomes during counselling session

CHILD/PARENT	RATIONALE	WHAT TO DO
Silence at start of session. Lack of eye contact	Inability to voice worries. Fear of naming that which concerns them most.	Remain silent for a while. Then say that it is sometimes difficult to know where to start. Ask what it is that is most difficult for them at that moment. Use gentle probing questions and remain focused on child parent during the silences.
Silence in the middle of the session	Child parent may be reflecting on what has just been said. May also have triggered off a difficult memory.	Be sensitive to the silence. After a while remark that you can see that they have been thinking quietly. Ask if they would like to share that thinking with you. Be aware of body language and mixed messages: i.e. child parent: 'Oh, I'm OK — its nothing really' said with crossed arms and legs and no eye contact.
Tears	Relief at being able to talk about concerns.	Pass the tissues and let the child parent cry.
Tears	Fear of what their new knowledge may mean	Pass the tissues. Ask what is happening in their head at this moment. What are they feeling in relation to this new knowledge?
Jokey, flippant remarks about having AIDS	Minimisation of real issue	Ask what 'having AIDS' might mean to them.
Inappropriate smiling	Can mask a very frightened child	Watch body language and check for mixed messages.
Smiling midway or at end of session	Relief at new understanding of issue	Smile back and ask them to tell you what they understand by what has just been said.
Sharing of new information relating to welfare of themselves re child sexual abuse	This usually means child is asking for help and is trusting you	Clarify this information. Ask if they would be willing to tell somebody else these new facts. Go slowly.
Sharing of new information relating to welfare of other children re child sexual abuse	As above	As above. Explain that you cannot help other child without their assistance.
Refusal to repeat information to social worker police	Fear of reprisal for themselves others by abusers	Explain as above. Offer to accompany child to social worker police. If all else fails, explain that you will have to tell somebody as, you have a duty to report this to Social Services and cannot keep this a secret. Take your time and go gently. There may be tears.

How to finish a session

When reaching the end of any session, whether it be preliminary, pre- or post test counselling, a short summary can clarify any points of uncertainty and round off the meeting. It may also be a useful way of checking that the child remembers this new information, and understands it. Practitioner:

> 'We're almost at the end of our time together today and I'm wondering whether you can tell me what you now understand about HIV infection and AIDS?'

The child may find it useful to make a list of all the information on a flipchart pad. This can then be taken away and looked at during the period of time needed for reflection and understanding prior to any other sessions. The next session should be at least one week later but not later than two weeks.

Pretest counselling

This should be the second session with the child and the practitioner can now begin to build on trust formed in session one.

A way of opening the pretest counselling session is to ask the child to tell you what they have remembered about HIV infection and AIDS. This again clarifies knowledge learned and helps evaluate the process of informed consent should testing take place.

Some questions for pretest counselling

What can you remember about how HIV is passed on?

What fluids is it passed from person to person in?

How is it not passed on?

How do you think you may have been infected with HIV?

What are you able to tell me about HIV antibodies?

What do you think a negative test would mean?

What do you think a positive test would mean to you?

What do you understand by the words 'risk activity'?

What is safer sex?

Who would you most want to tell if you were HIV positive?

What do you think they would say/do?

Would you want your parents to know the result of your test before you knew?

What do you understand about life insurance and mortgages?

What adult would you want to be present if the test were positive?

How would you want me to tell that adult?

These and the many more questions that the practitioner will develop with experience, enable the child to define their knowledge and the practitioner to clarify it.

If the child does opt for testing at the end of the session, it should be possible for blood to be taken for testing by the doctor who performed the medical examination after the alleged sexual abuse. This is preferable to most children than attending another clinic, and the child has the advantage of being seen by a known, sensitive face, thus reducing their anxiety and stress.

The doctor taking the blood will want to ask the child again to clarify their understanding of the test and what it means in order that informed consent to the test can be evaluated.

For the child who opts not to go ahead with HIV antibody testing, this will be their final session with the practitioner. Many children do opt out of testing, having decided that, for them, there would be little, or no advantage in having the test.

Whenever this option is chosen, it is just as important for the practitioner to discuss future relationships or other risk practices, as it would be if the child had had a test, regardless of result.

Post test counselling

Whatever the result of the test there will be a reaction (*see* chapter 10). If the test is negative then the practitioner will need to ascertain what the child understands by a negative result. It may be appropriate at this stage to discuss again and reinforce safer sexual or other practice. This will depend on the child's age and individual circumstances. Further testing in 12 weeks time may be necessary and the check-list questions from *pretest counselling* will need to be asked again by the practitioner and by the doctor who takes the specimen of blood.

If the test is positive do not underestimate the shock that this information will cause. Ensure that a psychiatrist/psychologist is on hand (even if not in the same room) and, if appropriate, the parent or named adult, whom you may already have informed.

If possible ask what the child's immediate concern is, then
IDENTIFY:
- What might be of help in dealing with that concern
- Who they may want to tell
- How they think they may tell them
- What being HIV positive means to them
- Whom they are going to turn to for support within their family unit

The child will need to meet the practitioner again, when the information has had time to be processed, for clarification of all issues. Meanwhile the practitioner needs to involve the paediatrician, and a professional who is able to provide a long term therapeutic relationship e.g. psychiatrist, psychologist, specially trained social worker (*see* Figure 3.13.1 in chapter 13).

Knowing when to refer to another professional is of utmost importance. The practitioner may have built up a relationship with the child which both may have difficulty in severing. However, other professionals will also build a relationship and it is in the child's best interest that they are being referred. Some counsellors will be in a position to refer to others and still remain the principal counsellor for the child, such as when involving doctors.

Despite the understandable hesitancy on the part of some professionals to counsel in this area, children and adults do find the counselling process a liberating experience. It provides a forum for naming their concerns, enabling them to begin to manage those concerns more effectively and make the transition from victim to survivor.

However, this book is not the definitive guide to counselling about HIV issues in child sexual abuse. It is merely an attempt to open up some issues for practitioners; clarify other issues; and also to provide a framework for good practice. It is offered as a tentative first step through the minefield to those who work in this difficult area, and recognise that children with worries about HIV have the right to honest information applied with sensitivity, humanity and commonsense.

References

Egan G, 1990 *The skilled helper: a systematic approach to effective helping* 4th edn. Brooks/Cole, California.

Resources

For the practitioner

AIDS, social representations, social practices. In Aggleton P, Hart G, Davies P (eds) 1989. Falmer Press.

Aggleton P, Homans H, Mojsa J, Watney S, Watson S, 1989 *AIDS: scientific and social issues.* Churchill Livingstone.

Aggleton P, Homans H, Mojsa J, Watson S, Waney S, 1989 *Learning about AIDS.* Churchill Livingstone.

Aggleton P, Horsley C, Warwick I, Wilton T, 1990 *AIDS working with young people* AVERT.

Allen I, 1987 *Education in sex and personal relationships.* Policy Studies Institute.

Bain O, Saunders M, 1990 *Out in the Open: A Guide for Young People Who Have Been Sexually Abused.* Virago Press.

Bancroft J, 1983 *Human sexuality and its problems.* Churchill Livingstone.

Bannister A, Barrett K, Shearer E (eds), 1990 *Listening to children: the professional response to hearing the abused child.* Longman.

Braun D, 1988 *Responding to child abuse: action and planning for teachers and other professionals.* Bedford Square Press.

The Charity Collective, 1983 *Taught not caught: strategies for sex education.* Learning Development Aids.

Clarke D, Underwood J, 1988 *Assertion training.* National Extension College.

Egan G, 1985 *Exercises in helping skills: a training manual to accompany the skilled helper.* Brooks/Cole, California.

Egan G, 1990 *The skilled helper: a systematic approach to effective helping* 4th edn. Brooks/Cole, California.

Holt J, Myers T, Quill D, Latham M, Oliver A, (eds) 1989 *Picking up the pieces: child sexual abuse and the juvenile justice system.* Hilltop Project's Practice Development and Publications Unit.

Honigsbaum N, 1991 *HIV/AIDS and children.* National Children's Bureau.

Miller D, 1987 *Living With HIV and AIDS.* Macmillan.

Saunders P, Farquhar C, 1991 *Positively primary: strategies for approaching HIV/AIDS with primary school children.* AVERT.

Scott P (ed), 1988 *National AIDS Manual.* N.A.M. Publications.

Useful organisations

Children's Legal Centre
20 Compton Terrace
London N1 2UN
Tel: 071-359 9392

Information sheets, booklets
on all aspects of children and
the law.

Haemophilia Society
123 Westminster Bridge Road
London SE1 7HR
Tel: 071-928 2020

Leaflets, booklets and advice
on living with HIV and
haemophilia.

IMMUNITY
260a Kilburn Lane
London W10 4BA
Tel: 081-968 8909

Leaflets, legal and welfare
advice and representation
around HIV/AIDS.

The MacFarlane Trust
PO Box 627
London SW1 0GQ
Tel: 071-233 0342

Charitable Trust, distributes
money provided by the
government to those who were
infected by HIV as a result of
treatment for haemophilia.

*Positively Partners and
Positively Children*
100 Shepperdess Walk
London N1 7JN
Tel: 071-738 7323

Counselling, advice, grants,
holidays and respite care.

The Terrence Higgins Trust
52/54 Grays Inn Road
London WC1X 8JU
Tel: 071-831 0330

THT offers a comprehensive
service which includes
counselling, education, welfare
and legal issues.

Developmental issues

Bee H, 1989 *The Developing Child* 5th edition. Harper Collins, New York.

Donaldson M, 1978 *Children's Minds*. Fontana, Glasgow.

Flavell J H, 1985 *Cognitive Development* 2nd edition. Prentice-Hall, Englewood Cliffs, New Jersey.

Gormly A V, Brodzinsky, 1989 *Lifespan Human Development* 4th edition. Holt Rheinhart and Winston inc, Florida.

Roberts M, Tamburrini J, 1981 *Child Development 0–5*. Holmes McDougall, Edinburgh.

Sylva K, Lund I, 1982 *Child Development. A First Course*. Grant McIntyre, London.

Index